Feed Your Genes Right

Feed Your Genes Right

Eat to Turn Off Disease-Causing Genes and Slow Down Aging

Jack Challem

WILEY

John Wiley & Sons, Inc.

Published by John Wiley & Sons, Inc., Hoboken, New Jersey
Published simultaneously in Canada

Design and composition by Navta Associates, Inc.

For general information about our other products and services, please contact our Customer Care Department within the United States at (800) 762-2974, outside the United States at (317) 572-3993 or fax (317) 572-4002.

Wiley also publishes its books in a variety of electronic formats. Some content that appears in print may not be available in electronic books. For more information about Wiley products, visit our web site at www.wiley.com.

Library of Congress Cataloging-in-Publication Data:

Challem, Jack.
 Feed your genes right : eat to turn off disease-causing genes and slow down aging / Jack Challem.
  p. cm.
 Includes bibliographical references and index.
 ISBN 978-0-471-77867-7
 1. Nutrition–Genetic aspects. 2. DNA damage–Prevention. 3. Diet in disease. I. Title.
 QP143.7.C48 2005
 613.2–dc22

2004024636

I dedicate this book to DeWitt Garrett, who first taught me about the health benefits of vitamins and nutrition.

CONTENTS

FOREWORD

The study of DNA in heredity and disease has led to a great many heady scientific discoveries and, ironically, to some humbling acknowledgments of ancient medical wisdom.

Scientists discovered nucleic acids, the general chemical building blocks of DNA (deoxyribonucleic acid) and genes, in the 1890s. Within several decades, biochemists and biologists had gained an impressive understanding of how nucleic acids were involved in heredity, and by 1950 experiments with bacteria had proven that DNA transmits inherited traits from one generation to the next.

Perhaps the single most dramatic event to ignite the imagination and enthusiasm of biologists was the 1953 discovery by James Watson and Francis Crick of the double-helix structure of DNA. All that remained, or so it seemed at the time, was to decipher and describe the genetic code in terms of its four-letter chemical alphabet.

But unraveling the details of DNA and its role in health and disease has turned out to be a far more complex and, at times, vexing process. As it turned out, the new millennium coincided with the complete decoding of the human genome, and this catalog of all human genes has led to many new insights into the function of DNA. Unfortunately, the promise of turning these discoveries into practical ways of preventing and treating disease has so far been disappointing. Cardiovascular diseases remain the leading cause of death in the United States and most of the developed world, while the scourge of cancer continues to take its relentless toll despite minor advances in treatment and prevention. Gene therapy has proven dangerous and difficult and has had few significant successes. Despite our current understanding of cancer-causing oncogenes and the details of how genes function, researchers have devised few new and effective therapies for cancer patients.

Quite surprisingly, the promise of improved treatment and prevention of human disease has emerged from an unexpected source: the study of nutrition. This was unanticipated for a couple of reasons. Despite the fact that two thousand years ago, Hippocrates, the father of Western medicine, wrote that food was our best medicine, this idea somehow came to be considered quaint rather than relevant. In addition, modern medicine has often derided and dismissed the role of nutrition in health.

However, increasing numbers of researchers and physicians have begun to acknowledge that the foods we eat lay the foundation for the biochemical milieu of our DNA. For example, the body's production of new DNA, required for health and healing, depends on the presence of many vitamins. The activity of DNA is further influenced by various nutrients' intersecting with genetically determined biochemical processes. And the progression of many diseases can often be influenced or ameliorated by careful adjustments in the intake of dietary nutrients.

This is a brave new world—and an exciting one at that—in the fields of both genetics and nutrition. But it has been many years in coming. An excellent example of the interaction of genetics and nutrition was my 1969 discovery of arteriosclerotic vascular disease in children with an inherited disease called homocystinuria. The most common form of homocystinuria is caused by a single abnormal gene, which programs the construction of the enzyme cystathionine beta synthase. This genetic defect results in elevated blood and urine levels of homocysteine, a toxic molecule now recognized in medicine as a risk factor for coronary artery disease and stroke.

The normal activity of the cystathionine beta synthase enzyme activity depends, humbly enough, on vitamin B_6. Approximately half of all children with this genetic condition respond favorably to large doses of vitamin B_6 with a dramatic lowering of homocysteine levels and a marked reduction in the risk of blood clots and cardiovascular disease. This is but one demonstration of how a genetic disease can be ameliorated by nutritional therapy.

In this important new book on genetics and human disease, the remarkably talented nutrition and health writer Jack Challem clearly explains the importance of nutrition and lifestyle factors in modifying the genetic underpinnings of many human diseases. He draws upon diverse yet authoritative sources to give reliable, sound, effective, and well-reasoned advice. The impressive advances in nutrition and biochemistry over the past several decades parallel the growing under-standing of the human genome and the genetic basis of human disease. The merging of these two fields sheds new light on the process of aging and the causes of human degenerative diseases.

Not only does *Feed Your Genes Right* explain the scientific understanding of nutrition and genetic disease, but also the sound, knowledgeable advice on treatment and prevention given is put into understandable and practical terms in an achievable program of prac-tical dietary improvement. Following the nutritional and lifestyle advice in this book will help prevent the degenerative diseases all too common in our twenty-first-century world.

—Kilmer S. McCully, M.D.
Author,
The Homocysteine Revolution and
The Heart Revolution

PREFACE

If you're like me, you want to maintain and perhaps improve your health, reduce your chances of developing disease, stay mentally sharp, stay at a normal weight, and remain physically active as you get older. But as I'm sure you've already discovered, there is no shortage of how-to health books or programs, frequently offering odd, counterintuitive, or contradictory advice.

How do you make sense of everything you hear?

Today, in the early years of the twenty-first century, medical research is dramatically shifting its focus. Instead of looking only at the physical or biochemical factors that lead to health problems, researchers are gaining a better understanding of the far-reaching roles genes play in determining the risk of disease. Now and in the years to come, the role of genes in health will strongly influence, and perhaps even dominate, recommendations for maintaining health and avoiding disease.

The truth is that your genes *do* play a fundamental role in health and disease. These tiny molecules, found in each one of your body's 70 trillion cells, contain biological instructions that orchestrate the functions of those cells and of your body as a whole. Your genes govern the activities of your heart, lungs, brain, and every other organ. The collective efforts of your genes determine how well your body functions—or malfunctions, as the case may be. Quite simply, when your genes do their job properly, you're in good health. When they don't, or can't, you are more likely to develop heart disease, cancer, and other diseases.

You have probably heard people say that "you've got the genes you were born with," suggesting that your health and risk of disease were sealed at birth. But contrary to popular opinion, genes are not rigid and inflexible determinants of your health, and your life is not merely an execution of some biological program beyond your control.

Instead, your genes possess extraordinary flexibility, which you can use to live a longer and healthier life. How is this possible? The reason is that genes do *not* function by themselves. Rather, *gene activity depends on a variety of nutrients as cofactors.* Nutrients provide the building blocks of genes, and they turn many genes on and off. Because you control what you put into your mouth, you can literally *feed your genes right* and gain tremendous health benefits. Or you can feed your genes all the wrong foods and suffer the unfortunate consequences. Vitamins and minerals (and many other nutrients as well) have always been essential cofactors for the normal functioning of your genes.

If these ideas seem strange or unfamiliar, rest assured. Research on the interactions between nutrition and genes is in step with many of the public-health recommendations you have heard over the years. For example, doctors have long urged the adoption of various dietary and lifestyle habits to reduce the risk of heart disease and cancer, such as eating more vegetables and fruit and exercising regularly. Nutrients work on multiple levels in the body, and ultimately they enable genes to function more efficiently, the way nature intended them to.

I first became interested in the health benefits of nutrition in 1969, when DeWitt Garrett, a college biology professor, made an intriguing off-the-cuff comment about vitamin supplements. The timing was serendipitous. I had recently been diagnosed with a cyst that my physician said would bother me for the rest of my life. About a week after I'd started to take vitamin supplements, my cyst drained and disappeared. I was impressed by the immediate and dramatic effect of the vitamins, and I have been taking them ever since. Looking back, I now realize that nutrient deficiencies likely interfered with the genes involved in healing the cyst, a situation that the vitamin supplements corrected.

It was not until the mid-1990s, however, that I started to see a clear connection between nutrition and genes. Bernard Rimland, an autism researcher, happened to tell me about a physician who had used large dosages of vitamins and other supplements to treat children with Down syndrome, a disorder caused by an irreversible genetic defect that leads to physical abnormalities and mental retardation. Rimland told me that the earlier children began taking the supplements, the more likely they would grow up with near-normal intelligence and appearance. Somehow, massive amounts of vitamins and other supplements managed to offset much of the genetic chaos of Down syndrome.

Hearing about the nutritional treatment of Down syndrome, I began to mull over whether we are "what we inherit." I had reason to be curious. My older brother had died from cancer at a relatively young age, and my parents had died after many years of failing health. I did not want to follow in their footsteps, at least if I didn't have to.

I mulled over a simple question: if vitamin supplements could undo a significant amount of the genetic damage done by Down syndrome, why couldn't vitamins and dietary changes improve other types of genetic defects or damage? It turned out that other people were thinking along the same lines. Researchers around the world were discovering that vitamins, such as vitamin E and the B vitamin folic acid, could reduce much of the cumulative genetic damage that occurs during the aging process and in many diseases.

Shortly afterward, I had an opportunity to experiment on myself. In 1997, at age forty-seven, I grappled with the fact that I was twenty pounds overweight and my blood sugar was creeping up toward prediabetic levels. I was slowly but steadily heading toward type 2 diabetes. For a health writer, this situation was, at the very least, embarrassing. But I was at a loss as to how to change it.

The solution came with advice from people who were more savvy than I was when it came to nutritional supplements and diet. A nutritionally oriented physician conducted a battery of blood tests and found that I was low in key minerals involved in managing blood sugar and insulin. So I started taking supplements of these minerals, including chromium, magnesium, and zinc. I also increased my intake of alpha-lipoic acid, a vitamin-like nutrient involved in regulating blood sugar and insulin levels. But supplements were not the entire solution. Two years later a nutritionist coached me on eating more wholesome foods as a way to lose weight and control my blood sugar.

By eating more nutritious foods, cutting out the all-too-convenient junk foods, and continuing to take certain nutritional supplements— what I now call feeding my genes right—I effortlessly lost twenty pounds and four inches from my waist in three months. I also found, a little later, that my blood sugar and insulin levels fell to well within normal ranges. Knowing what I do now, I understand that these changes helped turn off genes involved in overweight, inflammation, and diabetes.

All of these events were stepping-stones to a more serious examination of how nutrition influences the activity of genes and, in turn, overall health. With all the news reports about gene research and (so far exaggerated) promises of future gene therapies, most physicians and researchers have ignored a simple yet profound fact: our genes require many nutrients to do their jobs correctly, just as you and I need a good meal to feel up to doing *our* jobs.

Feed Your Genes Right is the result of both a personal and a professional quest, one that I am pleased to share with you. This book explains, in simple and nontechnical terms, how nutrition affects your genes and your risk of disease, regardless of whether you have inherited "good" or "bad" genes.

In Part I, I provide an overview of nutrition-gene interactions, explaining how genes become damaged and how they are capable of repairing themselves, so long as they receive proper nutrition. In Part II, I provide the Feed Your Genes Right Supplement Plan, which describes specific vitamins and vitamin-like nutrients needed for healthy genes. Part III covers dietary recommendations for maintaining healthy genes, explaining what you should and should not eat. Finally, Part IV describes how stress affects genes, suggests antistress nutrients you can take, and makes specific recommendations for reducing genetic damage that occurs in aging, heart disease, cancer, some inherited diseases, and many other conditions.

The bottom line of *Feed Your Genes Right* is that you do not have to wait years to apply the new and exciting discoveries of nutrigenomics, the science of nutrition and genetics. You can utilize existing knowledge to improve your health today and to set the stage for an active, healthy, and long life. I have incorporated these concepts in my own life, and you can, too.

Be healthy, and enjoy life!

ACKNOWLEDGMENTS

Many individuals have contributed in a variety of ways to my work on this book. I wish to thank Jack Scovil, my agent, and Tom Miller, my editor at John Wiley & Sons, for their support of this book and trust in my perspective and ideas. I also wish to thank Kimberly Monroe-Hill and Maureen Sugden for their careful editing of the manuscript.

I thank Sally Krusing for her enthusiasm in sharing her culinary experience, for helping me develop and test many of the recipes, and for reading and commenting on the manuscript.

I thank Bill Thomson, a friend and former editor of *Natural Health* magazine, for helping me refine many of my ideas and for his comments on the manuscript.

Many other people generously shared scientific and medical information through discussions and e-mails, and I am indebted to them. They include Craig Cooney, Ph.D.; Abram Hoffer, M.D., Ph.D.; Ronald Hunninghake, M.D.; James Jackson, Ph.D.; Peter Langsjoen, M.D.; Ali Langsjoen, M.S.; Chris Matthews, Ph.D.; Kilmer McCully, M.D.; David S. Moore, Ph.D.; and Hugh Riordan, M.D.

PART I

The Nutrition-Gene Connection

1

Your Genes Depend on Good Nutrition

Nurture is reversible; nature is not.
—Matt Ridley

Almost every week scientists announce the discovery of new genes that may influence our long-term risk of disease. The headlines and news stories tell us about genes that cause heart disease, Alzheimer's disease, breast cancer, prostate cancer, arthritis, diabetes, obesity, depression, schizophrenia, osteoporosis, and dozens of other diseases. As if we didn't already have enough to worry about, we now have to be concerned with whether we might be carrying any number of genetic time bombs.

We hear also that gene research may eventually lay the groundwork for new types of medical treatments. But until that time comes—and it will be years away at best—it's easy to feel victimized by our heredity. After all, we have been told for decades that our genes predetermine our health risks—genetic fatalism, so to speak—and that we can't do anything to change the genes our parents gave us.

Or can we?

The premise of *Feed Your Genes Right* corrects much of what you have previously heard. Your genes, of course, are the biological programs

3

that govern much of how your body functions or, as the case may be, *mal*functions and causes disease. But to the surprise of many scientists, recent research has revealed that your genes are not rigid, unchanging determinants of your health. Rather, you can improve your genetic heritage and the way your genes function. Quite simply, you can offset disease-causing genetic defects and age-related genetic damage with certain eating habits, nutritional supplements, and other lifestyle improvements.

As incredible as this may sound, the ability to modify the behavior of your genes forms a key concept in nutrigenomics, the scientific field that looks at how genes and nutrition interact. A large body of research clearly shows that the normal functioning of your genes depends on a good diet and a healthy lifestyle. By applying this research, you can foster healthier genes, slow your aging process (that is, feel and even look younger), and lower your risk of virtually every disease. *Feed Your Genes Right* explains exactly how you can do this, with easy-to-follow advice.

Is Nutrition All That Important?

People often seem surprised to hear that all of the foods they eat (not just fats and carbohydrates) affect their physical health, aging process, stress responses, and appearance. The truth is that the nutrients you consume are literally the building blocks—the bricks and mortar—of your body. Good nutrition provides a solid foundation for health. In contrast, poor eating habits make for a shaky foundation at best.

The importance of nutrition in health is hardly a new idea. More than two thousand years ago, Hippocrates, the father of Western medicine, wrote that food was our best medicine. Today many people understand that some foods, such as fish and vegetables, are healthy and reduce the risk of heart disease and cancer, whereas sugary soft drinks, doughnuts, and candy bars are unhealthy because they set the stage for obesity and diabetes.

What has changed since Hippocrates' time is our comprehension of the exact details and the full extent of how nutrition affects our health. Until relatively recently, researchers had a fairly general understanding of how some nutrients, such as vitamins and minerals, affect health. Scientists have now gained a new and profound knowledge of the specific ways that foods and individual nutrients affect the activity of genes and, consequently, the health of the entire body.

With this growing understanding of how nutrients and genes interact, it is now possible to determine whether you might need extra amounts of certain vitamins and minerals to stay healthy. Knowledge is power, of course, and you can use this knowledge to overcome genetic weaknesses and to reduce, slow, and sometimes reverse age-related genetic damage. The payoff? You can greatly improve your health, regardless of the genes you were born with. In a very real sense, you do not have to rationalize that a particular health problem "runs in my family," because you do not have to let the health problem run in *you*.

Your Genes Are Flexible, Not Fixed

Our genes consist of a microscopic double strand coil of deoxyribonucleic acid, better known simply as DNA. How are genes and DNA different? DNA is the equivalent of a biological dictionary. Genes use DNA to form an entire set of instructions guiding the behavior of each and every cell in our bodies.

This genetic program functions like the instructions written in a computer's operating system, or the underlying program that runs your computer. Our genetic program governs the entire organization and operation of our bodies, ensuring that nearly all people are born with arms, legs, lungs, a heart, and other organs. We often look like our parents because they were the source of our genes, passing along genetic programs that determined our hair, eye, and skin color.

However, your genes do far more than program your appearance. They orchestrate the creation of everything in your body, including fifty thousand proteins and tens of thousands of other biochemicals. Although many of your physical features (such as eye color) are fixed, the genes in charge of your day-to-day biochemical processes are not. Contrary to what many people have believed, genes are not destiny. Your genes provide tremendous flexibility in your long-term health, and you can use that flexibility to your advantage.

Your genes are always responding, in good or bad ways, to what you eat; to your emotions, your stresses, and your experiences; and to the nutritional microenvironment within each of your body's cells. If you maintain a particularly healthy genetic environment, your genes will function normally and you will age relatively slowly and be more resistant to chronic, degenerative diseases. If you maintain a less-than-healthy genetic environment, such as by smoking or eating large amounts of unhealthy foods, you will age faster and be more susceptible to disease.

The Promise of *Feed Your Genes Right*

By now you should realize that you do not have to live with health problems that make you feel less than your best and increase your risk of premature aging and disease. You also may be curious about the specific recommendations for feeding your genes right and improving your health.

As you read *Feed Your Genes Right*, you will discover how

- some inherited genes may be predisposing you to a variety of diseases that doctors commonly miss;
- age-related damage to your genes increases your risk of serious diseases, such as heart disease, Alzheimer's disease, and cancer, as well as saps your energy levels;
- nutritional deficiencies create biochemical bottlenecks, preventing genes from fulfilling their normal and intended functions;
- foods rich in sugars and refined carbohydrates boost levels of insulin, a hormone that alters gene activity and increases your risk of obesity, diabetes, heart disease, and cancer; and
- certain cooking habits can damage your DNA and accelerate the aging of your body.

But as the title suggests, *Feed Your Genes Right* is not just about what can go wrong with your genes and health. Instead this book emphasizes what you can do to protect your DNA and offset both inherited genetic weaknesses and age-related genetic damage. Most of this book explains how

- healthy, nutrient-dense foods, such as fish and vegetables, provide optimal nourishment for your genes and turn off many disease-promoting genes;
- some foods, such as kiwifruit, blueberries, and raspberries, actually help prevent and repair DNA damage;
- B vitamins help your body make and repair DNA and regulate the behavior of your genes, something that becomes especially important after age thirty;
- antioxidants, such as vitamins E and C, protect DNA from thousands of dangerous molecules each day;
- selenium, an essential nutrient, turns on genes that fight cancer cells; and

- vitamin-like nutrients, such as coenzyme Q10 and carnitine, counteract DNA-damaging molecules and boost your energy levels.

The take-home message of this book is really very simple: you can slow down your body's aging process, reduce your risk of chronic and catastrophic diseases, maintain high energy levels, stay sexually active, preserve a more youthful appearance, and remain mentally sharp as you reach middle and old age. You can do this by providing your genes with the best nutritional environment for their normal—and even optimal—functioning.

The key to accomplishing all of this, simple as it might sound, is eating nutritious foods, taking certain vitamins and other types of supplements, engaging in moderate physical activity, and limiting the harmful negative stresses in life. I've succeeded in doing these things myself, and I have known people in their seventies and eighties who look and feel decades younger than they really are by doing the same.

—⁓—

The Feed Your Genes Right Quiz:
Assessing Your Health and Risk of Disease

Your risk of disease is influenced by a variety of factors, including the genes you inherit from your parents and how your genes are shaped by the dietary and environmental factors unique to your life. This quiz assesses some of the risk factors affecting the health and function of your genes. Simply circle yes or no, depending on whether the statement applies to you.

Your Inherited Risk Factors

I am more than forty years old.	Yes	No
My father died of a heart attack before the age of fifty.	Yes	No
My mother died of breast or cervical cancer before the age of forty.	Yes	No
Some serious diseases, such as arthritis, cancer, diabetes, heart disease, obesity, or others, seem to run in my family.	Yes	No
I was born with a recognized birth defect, such as a cleft lip or a cleft palate, or I have been diagnosed with a genetic condition.	Yes	No

Explanation: Yes answers point to a risk of disease related to either inheritance or age-related genetic damage.

Your Current Health Status

I am a little overweight.	Yes	No
I am considerably overweight and so is (was) at least one of my parents.	Yes	No
My energy levels are not as high as I would like, and I often feel too tired to do the things I would like to do.	Yes	No
I have been diagnosed with glucose intolerance, insulin resistance, Syndrome X, or diabetes.	Yes	No
I have been diagnosed with some type of cardiovascular disease or cancer.	Yes	No
I regularly take two or more different medications for conditions my doctor has diagnosed.	Yes	No
The older I get, the more forgetful I seem to become.	Yes	No

Explanation: Yes answers indicate that your genetics, cell function, and metabolism have been compromised, most likely because of dietary or lifestyle habits. The more yes answers, the more seriously your genes and health have already been compromised.

Your Stress Levels

I am under a lot of stress at home, at work, or while commuting.	Yes	No
I have a lot of resentment or anger about things that are not the way they should be in my life.	Yes	No
I have not been in a long-term relationship for at least several years, or I am in a relationship that I do not find enjoyable and satisfying.	Yes	No
I tend to have a lot of "down" days or often feel depressed.	Yes	No

Explanation: Yes answers reflect a high level of stress, which can lead to an imbalance in brain chemistry and altered gene function in brain cells.

Your Dietary and Exercise Habits

I usually skip breakfast, or I just have something like coffee and a doughnut.	Yes	No
I do not like eating vegetables, and I do not eat them regularly.	Yes	No
I eat a lot of my meals in fast-food restaurants.	Yes	No
I make most of my meals at home by heating something from a box in the microwave oven.	Yes	No
I smoke cigarettes.	Yes	No

I drink spirits (hard liquor) or beer every day.   Yes   No

I am too busy or too tired to exercise regularly.   Yes   No

Explanation: Yes answers indicate that you are not providing a sound nutritional or lifestyle environment for your genes. Even if you are currently free of disease, you are experiencing accelerated genetic damage, which will set the stage for serious chronic disease.

To Finish the Quiz

Add up your yes answers. If you did not circle any yes answers at all, you are in great shape, have good eating habits, and have good family genetics. If you circled just a few yes answers, you may be thinking that it's nearly impossible to achieve a perfect score—and that this quiz is stacked against you. But it is not. Rather the quiz is designed to show how many heredity, dietary, and lifestyle factors can work against you and the health of your genes. Every person inherits some types of genetic weaknesses and acquires additional genetic damage each and every day of his or her life.

—m—

The Failure of Gene Therapy

You might be wondering whether it would be easier to wait for medicine to develop high-tech gene therapies to correct any genetic weaknesses you have or might develop as you age. The problem with that line of thinking is that you may be dead before such research produces any benefits for the majority of people.

The reason is that a lot of gene research has been misguided by wishful thinking and oversold to investors and the general public. For example, reports of a "breast-cancer gene," a "heart-disease gene," or an "obesity gene" suggest that a single faulty gene causes each of these diseases. If this were the case, it might be relatively easy to develop gene therapies. But the "one gene, one disease" view is overly simplistic. Only about 10 percent of women with breast cancer have one of the so-called breast-cancer genes. The truth is that only a very small number of people have "smoking gun" genes that predispose them to obesity, diabetes, heart disease, Alzheimer's disease, or other disorders.

Although you don't read about it very often, genetic research has clearly shown that degenerative diseases are actually "polygenic." That is, most diseases involve hundreds and sometimes thousands of genes that go awry. Up to 5,000 malfunctioning genes set the stage for cardiovascular disease, almost 300 wayward genes are involved in asthma, and 140 faulty genes contribute to the problem of failing memory. And with the complex interplay of 30,000 genes and 3 billion units of DNA, it may very well be impossible ever to design truly effective multigene therapies to treat common diseases.

Another problem is that despite billions of dollars of research, gene therapies have so far been an abysmal failure. In most instances they have simply failed to work, and sometimes patients have developed cancer or died from mysterious causes. For example, many researchers have used genetically modified viruses to deliver disease-treating DNA. In some human experiments, these viruses missed their target and instead attached to the wrong gene, causing leukemia. The consequences of manipulating genes are often unpredictable, largely because of their inherent complexity.

The massive research effort to identify genes and turn gene therapy into a marketable product has for the most part ignored how genes— just like the rest of your body—depend on proper nourishment. Many scientists have been forced to accept the fact that thirty thousand genes cannot by themselves account for the phenomenal complexity of the human body. It is now becoming clear that vitamins and other nutrients directly and indirectly serve as cofactors in gene activity, strongly influencing how genes function.

Granted, foods and nutritional supplements are low-tech and considerably less glitzy than the latest much-touted medical discovery. They may even strike some people as being like quaint folk remedies. But the science behind nutrition and genetics is solid, and nutrition has the advantage of helping without causing harm. The most sensible approach is actually a generic one: for the majority of people, it is to eat foods and take supplements that enhance normal gene function and reduce gene damage throughout the body.

In the next chapter, we will look at some of the ways that DNA becomes damaged, as well as at DNA's ability to repair itself.

2

DNA Damage, Aging, and Disease

Whether you believe in God or are an atheist, it is hard not to be emotionally moved by "the miracle of life." However life began on earth, whatever or whoever initiated it, the nature of life—a newborn baby or hatchlings in a bird's nest—inspires awe and respect. In a process that is repeated millions of times each day, a single cell multiplies into a huge collection of diverse cells, operating with a level of interactivity and complexity that science is only starting to grasp.

The miracle of life begins, physically, with DNA. This double strand of molecules, too tiny to see without the most powerful electron microscope, contains all the instructions that transform us from a fertilized egg into a full human being. DNA also contains the biological programs for making the thousands of proteins, hormones, and other biochemicals involved in facilitating normal growth and healing, maintaining a normal heartbeat, fighting infections, suppressing cancer cells, and performing thousands of other jobs in the body. DNA is the biological instruction manual that enables your body to function relatively smoothly twenty-four hours a day, like the most complex of factories.

Your DNA keeps you healthy and alive, so long as you provide it with a nutrient-rich environment. When your DNA starts to malfunction, you will age faster than you would otherwise, and your risk of disease will increase as well. The reason for this is that malfunctioning DNA cannot provide the correct instructions to your body's cells, such as those in the heart or kidneys, to perform their jobs. Similarly, cancers arise from damaged DNA that incorrectly instructs cells to multiply uncontrollably. If you are like me, you want to keep your DNA in the best possible shape, because it means staying as youthful and healthy as you can.

A Quick Explanation of DNA, Genes, and Chromosomes

We regularly hear or read about DNA, genes, and chromosomes. But what exactly are they, what do they look like, and what do they do? In simple terms they provide organization to the biological instructions that influence everything that happens in your body, from the color of your eyes to your inherited risk of heart disease.

If you were to scrape off a little bit of skin from your fingertip and look at it under a microscope, you would find that it is not a single clump of tissue. Rather, your skin consists of individual units called *cells*, which perform various jobs. Your entire body consists of approximately 70 trillion cells, which operate both independently and cooperatively.

Each cell contains a nucleus, or an obvious center. If you focused your microscope inside the nucleus, you would see your genetic instructions organized into twenty-three pairs of *chromosomes*.

By increasing your microscope's magnification, you would see that the forty-six chromosomes are divided into approximately thirty thousand segments called *genes*. Each gene contains the instructions for making (or "coding" for) a single protein or enzyme. These genetic instructions might be the equivalent of "color hair black," "produce testosterone," or "make hemoglobin."

Looking more closely, you would find that genes consist of double strands of *DNA* (the abbreviation for deoxyribonucleic acid). DNA forms the words in genetic instructions, and the typical gene contains approximately seven hundred DNA words.

Sharpening your focus even more, you would find that DNA strands consist of four smaller chemical units called *nucleotide bases*. These chemicals (adenine, cytosine, guanine, and thymine) form the chemical alphabet of DNA. A single cell in your body contains 3 billion DNA letters, roughly the same number of letters found in thirty-seven thousand copies of this book.

To make a protein or enzyme, DNA creates a strand of *RNA* (ribonucleic acid) and then transcribes its instructions onto it. RNA then uses these instructions to select the individual amino acids (which are found in protein-containing foods) needed to make a specific protein or enzyme. These proteins and enzymes form the foundation of thousands of biochemicals, from hormones to neurotransmitters, required for your body to function.

How Genes Turn On

Over the years many researchers have attributed great powers to genes, often suggesting that they predestine most aspects of your health and disease risk. But by themselves genes do absolutely nothing. They are simply sets of biological instructions that remain quiet until something prompts their activity.

Biologists describe the activation of genes as "gene expression." When a gene becomes "expressed," it turns on, and only then does it begin the process of creating a protein or enzyme. Genes can be turned on by any number of factors, including normal growth, injuries, healing, stresses, hormones, emotions, and infections.

The process of gene expression is analogous to how a factory receives and fills orders. It begins when a cell receives a chemical signal, which is akin to an order for a specific part. The order is directed to the gene in charge of producing the protein or enzyme needed for that part. After the protein or enzyme is made, vitamins, minerals, and other nutrients are used to complete the manufacturing process.

If an important manufacturing ingredient—such as a specific vitamin—is not present in adequate amounts, production stops and the order cannot be filled. In practical terms this means that your body might not be able to make new cartilage to cushion your knees or produce the neurotransmitter serotonin to reduce anxiety.

As another example, let's say that you are cooking dinner and you accidentally cut your finger with a knife. Almost instantly a variety of chemical signals alert the entire body to what has happened. Some of these chemical signals activate immune cells, such as white blood cells, which rush to the cut and attack infecting bacteria. Other signals turn on genes involved in healing. During the healing process, some skin cells start making copies of their DNA and then divide to create new cells. After the cut heals, all this activity subsides, because it is no longer needed.

Nutrients Help Activate Genes

For genes to remain healthy and functional—to be turned on or off when they are supposed to be—their constituent DNA must be fed the proper nutrients. This is a little different from what you have previously heard about nutrition. Most of us have been taught that we need nutrition to live, and we have learned that we need many specific nutrients, such as vitamin A for our eyes and calcium for our bones. But only recently have researchers begun to appreciate the details of how nutrition affects our DNA and genes.

Despite the frequent news reports about DNA, genes, and health, most people never hear that the body's production of DNA depends on the presence of certain vitamins. For example, you must have an adequate intake of vitamins B_3 and B_6 and folic acid to make DNA. (The role of these vitamins will be discussed further in chapter 5.) Low intake of any of these and other vitamins, a problem that is surprisingly common, reduces the production of DNA needed for new and replacement cells. If you cannot make new DNA, you will be left with only damaged, old, or malfunctioning DNA—giving your cells the wrong instructions.

Many other nutrients play important roles in normal DNA function as well. Zinc, an essential dietary mineral, forms fingerlike structures within in DNA. Similarly, selenium, another essential mineral, is needed by a key cancer-suppressing gene. These nutrients and others will be discussed in greater detail in chapters 4, 5, and 6. Throughout this discussion, one of the key ideas to remember is this: vitamins and many minerals (and many other nutrients as well) are absolutely essential for health. Part of the reason they are essential is that genes need them for normal functioning and resisting disease.

Proof of Principle: Folic Acid, Vitamin D, and Our Genes

In the 1960s Welsh scientists and physicians reported that pregnant women eating diets low in the B vitamin folic acid (found in leafy green vegetables) had a high risk of giving birth to infants with a serious birth defect called spina bifida. It took a number of years, but researchers eventually realized that some of the women had genetic weaknesses that interfered with how their bodies processed folic acid, thus increasing the risk of birth defects.

Scientific studies focused on the gene that made an enzyme crucial to the body's processing of folic acid. Subtle defects in this gene led to the creation of an inefficient enzyme, which in turn interfered with folic acid's essential role in making new DNA and cells for a growing fetus. Without ample folic acid, normal DNA and cell production failed, and a birth defect was almost inevitable. But the researchers also found that women who increased their consumption of folic acid (either through foods or supplements) overcame this genetic defect and gave birth to healthy babies. The extra folic acid didn't change the gene, but it did enable the enzyme to work harder.

In recent years researchers realized that either the same genetic defect *or* low levels of folic acid could interfere with DNA-building processes throughout the body and at any time (not just during gestation in women). It turned out that low intake of folic acid can set the stage for widespread genetic damage, premature aging, heart disease, Alzheimer's disease, and even some types of cancer. In each case adequate or extra amounts of folic acid help maintain normal gene function.

A similar story recently began unfolding with vitamin D. Many people inherit a defect in the gene responsible for managing vitamin D in the body. More than a dozen variations in this gene have been identified so far. Some variations increase the risk of the bone-thinning disease osteoporosis, and others boost a person's chances of developing cancer, diabetes, or multiple sclerosis. The scientific evidence suggests that increasing one's intake of vitamin D or spending at least fifteen minutes daily in the sun (which stimulates the body's own production of vitamin D) can overcome this genetic defect and reduce the risk of these diseases.

How Jerry Saved His Heart

Jerry, now age fifty-six, is alive and well and in exceptionally good health—thanks to the fact that he has used nutrition to offset a potentially fatal genetic defect.

Nearly all of the men in Jerry's family have died at relatively young ages. His paternal grandfather died of a heart attack at forty-six. Jerry's father died after suffering his second heart attack at age thirty-eight. And Jerry's older brother died after a stroke at age forty-two.

Several years ago genetic testing found that Jerry carried a subtle defect in the gene programming the construction of methylenetetrahydrofolate reductase (MTHFR), an enzyme needed for normal utilization of the B vitamin folic acid. Because of this defect, Jerry did not efficiently use the modest levels of folic acid found in his diet. As a result his blood levels of homocysteine, a major risk factor for heart disease, were extremely high—34 micromoles per liter of blood. It is very likely that other men in Jerry's family carried the same MTHFR polymorphism.

To offset the sluggish MTHFR enzyme created by the gene, a nutritionally oriented physician recommended that Jerry take a daily high-potency B-complex vitamin supplement containing 800 mcg of folic acid. She also suggested that Jerry eat more vegetables and fewer high-carb and high-fat fast foods. Literally fearing for his life, Jerry also began exercising regularly and adopted stress-reduction habits, such as meditation, to deal with work-related pressures.

Today Jerry is a paragon of cardiovascular fitness. His homocysteine and blood-fat levels are normal, about 7 micromoles per liter of blood. In addition, his blood pressure is normal, and a treadmill test recently found him to be exceptionally fit.

Some Common Genetic Diseases

All degenerative diseases entail some type of impairment of DNA and gene activity. For example, some types of DNA damage are inherited and cause specific diseases, such as sickle-cell anemia. Cancer results from DNA damage that totally rewrites normal genetic instructions. As you get older, you acquire increasing amounts of genetic damage that affect your body's outward appearance and how well the interior of your body functions.

Aging. Although aging is not generally considered a disease, it possesses the genetic hallmarks of a disease: progressive damage to DNA that increases the risk of developing diseases. For example, wrinkled skin reflects underlying DNA damage to skin cells.

Cancer. Many different factors strongly influence the risk of developing cancer, but some people inherit unstable genes that increase susceptibility to cancer. For example, low activity of the p53 cancer-suppressing genes can increase the risk of many types of cancer. More often, however, random mutations to DNA can reprogram gene function, leading to normal cells' becoming cancerous.

Celiac Disease. This inherited disease causes a total intolerance of gluten, a family of proteins found in wheat and many other grains. The intolerance, which is somewhat like an allergy, commonly leads to an abnormal immune response centered in the gastrointestinal tract and causes poor nutrient absorption.

Coronary Artery (Heart) Disease. Although strongly influenced by diet and emotional stress, coronary artery disease can also be influenced by specific genes. For example, the APOE E4 gene promotes the accumulation of cholesterol, and some versions of the MTHFR gene can lead to elevated blood levels of homocysteine, which damages blood-vessel walls.

Favism. This intolerance to fava beans results from a genetic variation that interferes with the body's ability to break down toxic substances. As a consequence, two naturally occurring substances (vicine and divicine) in fava beans are toxic to people with this genetic trait.

Hemophilia. This disease, which prevents the normal clotting of blood, is caused by a genetic defect that impairs the body's use of vitamin K.

Hemochromatosis. This condition is caused by a genetic variation that interferes with regulatory mechanisms involved in iron absorption. People with hemochromatosis absorb too much iron, which can increase the risk of heart disease and other disorders.

Mitochondrial Myopathies. These conditions, which severely affect energy levels, result from defects in the DNA programming of energy production in cells. Because of these defects, people with mitochondrial myopathies cannot efficiently produce energy and suffer from extreme weakness and exhaustion.

Phenylketonuria. This condition results from a genetic defect in an enzyme that prevents the conversion of phenylalanine to tyrosine, both important amino acids. Symptoms affect the nervous system and include seizures and psychiatric disorders.

Pyroluria. Some people are genetically predisposed to excrete elevated levels of kryptopyrrole, which also depletes vitamin B_6 and zinc. The condition, called pyroluria, is found in many schizophrenic patients. Low levels of vitamin B_6 impair the synthesis of serotonin and many other neurotransmitters, so depression and moodiness may be other common symptoms. White spots on fingernails are a sign of zinc deficiency.

Sickle-Cell Anemia. In ancient times sickle-cell anemia, which distorts the shape of red blood cells, provided some protection against malaria. However, its symptoms include pain and a sharply increased risk of cardiovascular disease. It is most common in people of African descent.

How Too Much Iron Weighed Down Michael's Health

Michael, in his mid-thirties, was experiencing inexplicable physical symptoms. His skin was darkening, his knee joints were aching, and his interest in sex had practically vanished. The half-dozen physicians he had consulted could not come to a single diagnosis, and they suggested an array of treatments, including antiinflammatory drugs, testosterone patches, and antidepressant medications. One even suggested Michael spend less time in the sun, though he never was outdoors long enough to get a sunburn, let alone a tan.

Increasingly frustrated, Michael made an appointment with yet another physician. But this one had a hunch about the underlying cause of his health problems. Over the next several weeks, she ordered two different tests for his blood iron levels and then a test for a mutation in the HFE gene. Both tests came back positive. She diagnosed Michael with hemochromatosis, an inherited disease in which the body stores abnormally large amounts of iron.

Although iron is an essential nutrient, high levels can be dangerous and lead to a variety of seemingly disparate, difficult-to-diagnose symptoms. Untreated, hemochromatosis can lead to liver cancer, diabetes, heart failure, and premature death.

Michael's physician followed standard medical practice in treating hemochromatosis. She asked him to make weekly appointments for "serial phlebotomies"—medically sanctioned bloodlettings. Iron overload can be prevented by regularly drawing off a pint of blood. In addition, Michael consulted with a nutritionist, who recommended that he avoid iron-fortified grain products (such as breads and pastas) and iron-containing nutritional supplements.

Michael was lucky to be diagnosed early enough to reverse his symptoms. Over the next few months, all his symptoms began to subside.

How DNA Becomes Damaged

DNA damage occurs in a variety of ways, with the consequences interfering with the normal activity of our genes. The most common causes of damage include free radicals, replication errors in DNA, and transcriptional errors in DNA.

Aging is the most visible sign of ongoing DNA damage. Wrinkled skin reflects damage to the DNA and other structures of skin cells. Similar age-related DNA damage occurs in all organs, though at different rates, increasing our risk of degenerative diseases.

Free Radicals and DNA Damage

The most widely accepted theory of aging is based on the idea that unstable molecules called free radicals damage DNA. Free radicals form in the body as a by-product of the processes that break down food for energy, fight infections, and detoxify hazardous chemicals. They are also found in pollutants, such as automobile exhaust, cigarette smoke, copy machine fumes, and other types of air pollution. Still more free radicals are generated when tissues are exposed to radiation, such as ultraviolet rays in sunlight or the ionizing radiation of an X-ray.

Most free radicals are actually oxygen atoms, found in the air we breathe. Oxygen atoms become free radicals when they lose (or occasionally gain) one electron in what is normally a pair of electrons. To restore the equilibrium of two electrons, free radicals react with and steal an electron from any nearby molecule in a process called oxidation. The effect is somewhat like a row of falling dominoes, with one free radical being created after another, leaving large numbers of damaged molecules in their wake. Oxidation is what also causes iron to rust or silver to tarnish. In the human body, common targets of free-radical oxidation include fats, sugars, proteins, and DNA.

Your body accumulates free-radical damage throughout your lifetime. In fact, each cell in your body suffers an estimated ten thousand free-radical "hits" daily. Dr. Denham Harman, who conceived the free-radical theory of aging, has explained that most people stay ahead of this damage through efficient repair of DNA and other molecules until about age twenty-seven. After that point free-radical damage starts to accumulate faster than DNA can repair it.

While free-radical damage accumulates, it generally affects DNA in a random fashion. For example, free-radical damage from cigarette smoking concentrates in the lungs, where DNA mutations will increase the risk of cancer. But these free radicals also affect the heart and all other organs. The random nature of free-radical damage explains, at least in part, why one smoker might develop cancer while another suffers a heart attack.

Energy Production—the Major Source of Free Radicals

Nearly all the free radicals in the body are produced in mitochondria, microscopic structures in cells that break down food molecules for energy. During this process free radicals oxidize, or burn, glucose and fats much the way a car burns gasoline.

Luckily, most of these free radicals are held in chemical reactions within the mitochondria. However, some free radicals do leak out, and one of the first things they target is mitochondrial DNA. Mitochondria contain their own DNA (separate from the DNA in a cell's nucleus), which provides many of the genetic instructions for breaking down glucose and fats for energy.

When free radicals damage mitochondrial DNA, energy production becomes less efficient, leading to the leakage of increasing numbers of free radicals and still more damage to mitochondrial DNA. As these free radicals migrate, they also damage DNA in the cell nucleus, as well as fats, sugars, and proteins in cells, interfering with other cell functions. Many researchers believe that free-radical damage to mitochondria lies at the root of the entire aging process, which will be discussed further in chapter 4.

Inherited Mitochondrial DNA Defects

Many of the insights into mitochondria, DNA damage, and energy originated with studies of people with inherited or congenital diseases called mitochondrial myopathies. (Myopathies are diseases that affect muscle cells.) People with mitochondrial myopathies have damaged or missing segments of mitochondrial DNA, which reduces their body's production of energy. Because heart, skeletal-muscle, and brain cells have the highest concentration of mitochondria, these tissues are typically the ones most affected.

Symptoms of mitochondrial myopathies include extreme physical and mental fatigue. Droopy eyelids are also a common sign of these disorders. Symptoms often appear during infancy or early childhood and continue through adulthood. It is common for people with mitochondrial myopathies to feel totally exhausted after walking just a short distance. Poor concentration and low brain-wave activity may also be signs of some mitochondrial myopathies, and sometimes the damage is severe enough to result in mental retardation.

How Suzanne Fixed Her Energy Problems

Suzanne had felt weak and "foggy-brained" for as long as she could remember. As a child she had no energy or stamina for athletic activities, and as an adult, just walking around a grocery store left her feeling exhausted. Friends often kidded Suzanne, calling her "the ultimate couch potato" because sprawled on the sofa seemed like her most natural position.

At age twenty-six, Suzanne started to develop droopy eyelids and a slight tremor in her left arm, and she went to a neurologist for an exam and tests. The doctor arranged for a muscle biopsy, which was used to analyze Suzanne's mitochondrial DNA. The tests found that she had probably been born with damage to her mitochondrial DNA. She was diagnosed with a mitochondrial myopathy.

By pinpointing the specific location of the mitochondrial DNA damage, Suzanne's physician was able to recommend an appropriate treatment. He suggested that she take several supplements, including vitamin B_2, coenzyme Q10, and alpha-lipoic acid, all of which are involved in energy production. Suzanne's energy levels increased slowly, and several months after taking these supplements, her improved stamina has allowed her to enjoy more activities with her friends and family.

Acquired Mitochondrial DNA Damage

Interestingly, age-related accumulation of free-radical damage to mitochondrial DNA is very similar to what occurs in people born with mitochondrial myopathies. This explains, at least in part, why weakness and fatigue are commonly part of old age.

Although mitochondrial DNA damage is extensive in the elderly, significant damage can also occur at younger ages. One well-known case involves Greg LeMond, the bicycle racer who won two world championships and the Tour de France three times. Plagued with a variety of health problems, LeMond was diagnosed at age thirty-two with a mitochondrial myopathy. It was very unlikely that he was born with such mitochondrial damage, because it would have prevented him from excelling at bicycle racing. However, strenuous exercise generates large numbers of free radicals, and LeMond's intensive exercise (possibly without appropriate nutritional support) may have damaged his mitochondrial DNA.

A catastrophic loss of cellular energy production in mitochondria is also a factor in cardiomyopathy and heart failure, diseases of the heart muscle (as opposed to the more common coronary artery disease, which involves a blockage in key arteries). Heart cells require enormous amounts of energy to beat an average of 70 times a minute, 10,000 times a day, and 37 million times a year. All this energy must be generated by mitochondria in heart-muscle cells. While cardiomyopathy and heart failure sometimes result from damage to mitochondrial

DNA, these diseases may also result from low levels of the vitamin-like nutrients involved in energy production. These nutrients include co-enzyme Q10, alpha-lipoic acid, carnitine, ribose, and creatine (all of which will be discussed in chapter 4).

Some Nutrients That Protect DNA and Genes

Every nutrient directly or indirectly affects the health and performance of DNA and genes. The genetic roles of some nutrients, such as folic acid, vitamin D, and zinc, are well understood. The roles of others, such as carotenoids and flavonoids, are only now emerging. The following is a list of the most important nutrients affecting DNA and genes:

VITAMINS

Vitamin A. Influences the growth of cells and their differentiation into specialized cells.

B-Complex Vitamins. Play diverse roles in DNA synthesis, repair, and regulation.

Vitamin C. Enables generic stem cells to become specialized heart cells; it is also needed in energy-generating chemical reactions and the formation of proteins.

Vitamin D. Performs diverse hormonelike functions affecting bone density, immunity, and cancer risk.

Vitamin E. Protects DNA from free-radical damage and also helps regulate some genes.

VITAMIN-LIKE NUTRIENTS

Alpha-Lipoic Acid. Plays key roles in the production of energy and, as an antioxidant, in protecting DNA from damage.

Coenzyme Q10. Has a major role in producing energy in mitochondria.

Carnitine. Needed to transport fats into mitochondria so they can be burned for energy.

Carotenoids. A family of plant-based antioxidants that affect the activity of many genes; they also suppress a gene involved in skin inflammation.

Flavonoids. A large family of plant-based antioxidants; the flavonoid quercetin binds with DNA and may protect it against cancerous changes.

N-Acetylcysteine. Regulates many genes and also protects them from free-radical damage.

MINERALS

Chromium. Essential for the body's use of the hormone insulin, which influences genes involved in fat- and muscle-cell production.

Selenium. Needed for the normal functioning of the p53 cancer-suppressing gene.

Zinc. Provides key structural components, known as zinc fingers, to many genes.

DNA Mistakes during Cell Replication

Your body makes new cells when you are growing up, during the healing of injuries, and when old cells stop functioning or die and must be replaced. During cell replication, DNA makes a copy of itself, with the copy becoming part of the new cell.

The accuracy of DNA replication is exceptional—far better than that of the best typist—but it is not perfect. The replicated DNA may look virtually identical to the original, but typographical errors form in the chemical letters making up DNA.

These mistakes, or mutations, change a cell's programming, usually affecting it in a negative way. Most DNA mutations age our cells—and little by little our entire bodies—eventually making us more prone to organ dysfunction and disease. Furthermore, these mutations increase each time a cell makes a copy of itself, with errors leading to still more errors. That is why a fifty-year-old woman looks different from a twenty-year-old woman—the former has more DNA mutations.

We don't see the consequences of these mutations in the short term, but we do over a period of years. For example, you may not notice sun damage to your skin (reflecting underlying damage to skin-cell DNA) from one day to the next, but you will see changes to your skin over ten or twenty years.

DNA Errors during Transcription

During DNA transcription, the information encoded in specific genes is transferred to RNA, which then uses the information as a template for creating specific proteins or enzymes. These proteins and enzymes consist of chemicals known as amino acids. When you eat fish, chicken, eggs, or other protein-containing foods, the protein is broken down into amino acids in the digestive tract. The amino acids are subsequently delivered to cells and ultimately reassembled, following DNA instructions, into new proteins.

Problems occur when various amino acids are not present during transcription. If a needed protein or enzyme cannot be created, its absence may have enormous repercussions, such as low levels of the neurotransmitter serotonin and resultant depression.

Even when DNA transcription occurs with reasonable accuracy, other obstacles can prevent the production of proteins. For example, overcooking proteins creates substances known as advanced glycation end products, or AGEs. Like free radicals, AGEs easily damage DNA. There are ways to reduce production of AGEs, and these will be discussed in chapter 5.

Erik's Leukemia: Diffusing a Genetic Time Bomb

Erik, a physician, didn't know that he carried a genetic time bomb in his body.

One night in 1996, he felt nauseated and woke up with an elevated temperature and a pain in the side of his chest. His wife drove him to the hospital, where tests found that his white blood cell count was four times above normal. He was diagnosed with acute myelogenous leukemia, and the prognosis was chilling: without immediate treatment he would live no more than a few days. With treatment the odds were that he would not live much longer.

Erik was familiar with and had used nutritional therapy in his own medical practice, but he knew that it took time to work. With no time to spare, he decided to undergo conventional chemotherapy and tried to emotionally brace himself for the painful side effects. As best he could, because of regular vomiting, he took 10 grams of vitamin C, 400 IU of vitamin E, 500 mg of vitamins B_1 and B_6, and other supplements daily.

The chemotherapy bought Erik the time he needed, and after several weeks he increased the dosages of some supplements and added others, such as coenzyme Q10, to his regimen. As his leukemia went into remission and his white blood cell count normalized, he reduced the dosages of his supplements.

Erik beat overwhelming odds against him. A year after his

diagnosis, he was strong enough to resume his medical practice. After two years, a rare length of survival for this type of cancer, his doctors told him he had a 98 percent probability of remaining healthy for another three years. After that, he was venturing into medically unknown territory.

Now, in 2005, more than nine years after his initial diagnosis, Erik remains well. He attributes his long-term recovery to the benefits of high-potency nutritional supplements, many of which he still takes. Meanwhile, he focuses on his medical practice. "I have found it to be so rewarding to be able to concentrate on the problems of others rather than on my own fears for the future," he says.

How DNA Can Repair Itself

Like a publishing company, DNA also has proofreaders to catch and correct typographical errors in our genes. These proofreaders are enzymes that travel up and down the double strands of DNA, comparing one strand to another and excising and replacing incorrectly copied sections.

DNA-repair enzymes have their jobs cut out for them. More than ten thousand DNA bases in each cell break down each day just from normal body heat. Without DNA-repair enzymes, you would age much faster and would experience a much higher risk of cancer. To function, many of these enzymes depend on the presence of B vitamins, which will be discussed in chapter 5.

DNA-Repair Enzymes

The body has more than a dozen types of DNA-repair enzymes, but three appear to be the most important. *Mismatch-repair enzymes* correct mistakes made when DNA is copied during cell replication. These enzymes literally cut out and replace the errors. *Transcription-coupled repair enzymes* fix DNA errors during the transcription process, helping to prevent interruptions in the production of proteins and enzymes. *Nucleotide-excision repair enzymes* fix DNA that has become damaged, such as by free radicals.

The degree of accuracy in proofreading and correcting DNA mistakes is exceptional, but it is not perfect. Damage to a single strand of DNA is relatively easy to repair, but identical damage to both DNA strands is difficult to correct, because the repair enzyme then does not have reliable DNA to use as a model to follow.

A person's DNA-repair efficiency can have a powerful bearing on cancer risk. In a study published in the *Journal of the National Cancer Institute*, researchers found that women with breast cancer consistently had faulty DNA-repair processes. In contrast, only a small percentage of healthy women had poor DNA-repair processes. Women with a high risk of developing breast cancer were five times more likely to have sluggish DNA-repair mechanisms.

RNA Repair Enzymes

Until very recently RNA was considered little more than a simple messenger, transferring the information of DNA to create proteins and enzymes. Studies have now found that short strands of RNA, called microRNAs, help regulate cell growth.

RNA also plays a major proofreading role during DNA transcription. According to recent research, strands of "RNA interference" scan DNA for mutated genes. When RNA interference identifies a mutant gene, it signals other repair enzymes to come in and remove it.

Limitations of DNA Repair

Some people seem to be particularly prone to unstable DNA. This lack of structural stability can increase the risk of DNA mutations and cancer. In addition, some environmental contaminants, such as cadmium, directly interfere with normal DNA-repair processes. Also, aging cell membranes, which are basically the exterior and interior walls of cells, can prevent DNA-repair enzymes from moving from one part of a cell to another where they are needed.

Still, every person has a tremendous capacity for DNA repair, and you can enhance your ability to repair and maintain healthy DNA. Your DNA-proofreading and -repair enzymes depend in large part on the B vitamins. Antioxidants, such as vitamins E and C, can help protect DNA from damage. (We will discuss these vitamins in more detail in chapters 5 and 6.) There is compelling scientific support for using these vitamins to shore up the body's DNA-repair enzymes.

In the next chapter, we will consider how both longer life spans and modern eating habits have placed unprecedented stresses on genes, leading to their malfunction and hence to a greater risk of diseases.

3

Conflicts between Ancient Genes and Modern Foods

Despite the well-known relationships between poor eating habits and the risk of many common diseases, such as obesity, diabetes, heart disease, and cancer, most of us do not pay much attention to the quality of the food we eat. We do not usually associate food with how we feel from day to day, let alone with our long-term risk of disease. Nor do most of us realize that behind the more visible signs of health and disease, the foods we consume affect the activity of our genes.

All too often we eat to satisfy hunger pangs or cravings, instead of seeking good nutrition to maintain our health and, in the context of this book, normal or optimal gene function. We will often pick up a quick drive-through meal or pop a package into the microwave oven, because we have not allowed ourselves time to prepare a more wholesome meal. After we eat, we feel better for having quenched our immediate hunger, but many of the serious health consequences are usually years away, preventing us from connecting our eating habits with health.

Considerable research now points to specific ways that nutrients can positively affect genes and how we can put this information into practice. These boil down to three key areas that will be discussed at greater length subsequently:

1. Many of the individual nutrients a person routinely eats (or does not eat) directly affect the functioning of genes, which in turn influences both the daily sense of well-being and the long-term risk of serious disease.
2. Both inborn genetic weaknesses and age-related acquired genetic damage can be largely offset through the use of supplemental vitamins and other nutrients, fostering the optimal performance of our genes and overall biochemistry.
3. Research in several scientific disciplines, including the fields of nutrition, cell biology, molecular biology, and nutritional anthropology, points to particular eating habits and nutritional supplements that can enhance gene function in most people.

However, before turning to practical nutritional recommendations to enhance gene function, we must briefly consider the context—that is, our genetic and dietary heritage. This chapter focuses on some of the ways that modern eating habits and lifestyles have created new and unnatural stresses on our genes. It also provides a dietary framework for getting the most out of our genes.

The Genetic Downside of Living Longer

Most people would like to live a very long time, but, surprisingly, there are genetic consequences in doing so. One of the most significant consequences of living longer is having more time to acquire free-radical damage to our genes, resulting in an increased likelihood of developing chronic degenerative diseases.

To explain, until about ten thousand years ago, the average human life expectancy was approximately thirty years. Even as recently as 1900, most people in the United States lived only an average of fifty years, and the leading cause of death was infection. Today the average life expectancy is almost seventy-six years for American men and almost eighty years for American women. Over the past century, life expectancy in most other Westernized nations has increased significantly as well.

Instead of dying from extreme physical hardships, injuries, or infections at relatively young ages, most of us now live long enough to die from diseases related to long-term, cumulative DNA malfunctioning damage, such as heart disease, cancer, and Alzheimer's disease. If medicine somehow reduced deaths from these diseases, another disease would emerge as the leading cause of death. After all, we *will* die of something.

This discussion is not intended to be either wry or pessimistic. Rather it begs a very important question: what can we do to slow the inevitable genetic damage that develops during our longer lives? The answer is that we must take conscious steps to maintain the health of our genes.

For example, we know that smoking cigarettes and drinking large amounts of alcohol accelerate gene damage, the aging process, and the risk of various diseases. But we often forget that the opposite is also true—that we can slow down the age-related accumulation of DNA damage. Eating healthy foods, taking certain nutritional supplements, engaging in regular physical activity, and limiting psychological and emotional stresses all work to preserve and maintain normal or enhanced gene function. While these health recommendations might sound familiar, the rationale behind them and the specific suggestions in *Feed Your Genes Right* differ from those in other health books.

Ancient Genes, Modern Diet

Many modern health problems result from what amounts to a collision between our ancient genetics and modern highly processed foods. These foods, which include the vast majority of packaged products sold in supermarkets as well as fast foods, have undergone substantial modification from their original form, and they bear little nutritional resemblance to what people ate in the past.

As a result, our genes are routinely exposed to "genetically unfamiliar foods," and they respond abnormally, such as by triggering chronic inflammatory reactions. The solution is to bring our current eating habits more into line with our genetic requirements. This change might initially seem a bit daunting, but it is actually relatively easy to accomplish.

To figure out what we should eat for normal gene function and a relatively healthy and long life, it is useful to understand the nutritional environment that coexisted with and helped shape our genes over many years. For instance, we know that human beings and other mammals developed in *nutrient-dense* environments. In other words, nearly every calorie consumed came with relatively large amounts of vitamins, minerals, proteins, and healthy fats but relatively little starch (carbohydrate) and no pure sugars.

Nutrient-Dense Foods

So what exactly did early humans eat in the distant past? Dr. S. Boyd Eaton of Emory University and Loren Cordain, Ph.D., of Colorado State University have conducted extensive research on ancient hunter-gatherer diets, which is what all humans once consumed. People hunted wild animals for meat and foraged for edible plants. If they lived near an ocean, lake, or river, they likely caught and ate fish and other types of seafood as well. The relative percentages of animal foods versus vegetable foods varied from culture to culture, but, interestingly, no society was entirely vegetarian. Many ancient diets were extraordinarily diverse, including up to a hundred different types of plant foods, as well as scores of land animals, many species of fish, and wild bird eggs.

As varied as these ancient diets were, they all shared the common characteristic of nutrient density. People rarely if ever consumed "empty calories" largely devoid of other nutrients, as we often do today with various types of sugars, refined starches, very fatty foods, and alcohol.

So, over many years, nutrient-dense foods helped shape the structure and function of human genes. At the same time, our genes became dependent on foods containing relatively large amounts of vitamins and minerals but relatively small amounts of carbohydrate calories from starches and sugars. Around ten thousand years ago, human eating habits started changing with the advent of agriculture, which led to substantial increases in carbohydrate and sugar intake.

The consumption of nutritionally empty carbohydrates and sugars has accelerated greatly over the past hundred years and especially over the past thirty years, with the popularity of fast-food restaurants, convenience and microwave foods, soft drinks, and thousands of snack items on supermarket shelves. Today 80 percent of the carbohydrate calories consumed in the United States supply few nutrients besides sugars and refined starches.

How Are Ancient and Modern Diets Different?

Ancient and modern diets differ in many ways. Here are a few examples of those differences:

* *Vitamins and Minerals.* With the exception of sodium (in salt), ancient humans consumed two to six times higher levels of most vitamins and minerals.

- *Protein.* Ancient protein consumption ranged from 19 to 35 percent of total calories and sometimes up to 50 percent. Today protein accounts for about 15 percent of all calories.
- *Fats.* Human diets once provided 38 to 58 percent of calories as fat, compared with 34 percent today. However, the type of fat was substantially different. Ancient peoples consumed about equal amounts of omega-6 and omega-3 fats, but today the ratio is about 30:1 in favor of omega-6 fats. Both families of fats influence gene activity and provide biochemical building blocks for the immune system. The omega-6 fats, found in corn oil, safflower oil, and other common cooking oils, promote inflammation. In contrast, the omega-3 fats, found in fish and grass-fed livestock, are antiinflammatory.
- *Carbohydrates and Fiber.* Ancient carbohydrates were found in vegetables, fruits, nuts, and seeds, not in grain-based food products (such as breads and pastas). In addition, these carbohydrates were part of a fiber matrix that buffered their absorption. In the past, people consumed about 100 grams of fiber daily; today it is about 20 grams.

Different Diets, Different Genetic Messages

By comparing ancient and modern diets, it becomes clear that modern refined and processed foods are very different from the foods that originally nurtured our genes. This difference—the incompatibility of modern foods with ancient genes—accounts for much of the current prevalence of degenerative diseases. But what, you might ask, are some of the specific genetic consequences of a diet incompatible with our biological heritage?

When we consume a diet built around foodstuffs that did not exist until recently, our ancient genes receive unfamiliar chemical signals. Sometimes they misinterpret these signals and, not surprisingly, respond abnormally. For example, diets high in sugars and refined starches, which are relatively new components of human diets, turn on genes that promote inflammation, obesity, and diabetes.

The response of genes to genetically unfamiliar foods is nearly always abnormal. It is as if they are struggling to interpret and respond to a foreign language. Imagine your genes as American tourists trying to follow travel directions in Greek, and it might be somewhat comical. But there is nothing funny when genes misunderstand chemical messages and their reactions then set the stage for chronic disease.

Excess Carbohydrates Alter Gene Function

The significant difference between past and present eating habits becomes clear in a simple comparison. Twenty thousand years ago, people hunted and foraged for their food, eating lean meats, seafood, and organic (pesticide-free) vegetables that resembled our modern kale, rose hips, and crabapples. The diet could be described as high in protein, relatively low in saturated fat, and high in nonstarchy (low-carbohydrate) vegetables and fruits. Hunter-gatherers also had to be physically active to obtain food, which stimulated genes to increase the number of muscle cells and the number of mitochondria within muscle cells. Under these circumstances obesity was rare, if it occurred at all.

Today many people still forage, but they do so by choosing highly refined and processed items from the menus of McDonald's, Burger King, Taco Bell, and other fast-food restaurants. A burger, fries, and a soft drink provide mostly sugars, other refined carbohydrates, and saturated and trans fats but little quality protein and few vitamins and minerals. Such a meal is calorie-dense and carbohydrate-dense but not nutrient-dense.

Eating large quantities of empty carbohydrate calories—the average person now consumes 150 pounds of sugars each year—raises glucose levels, which in turn increase the secretion of insulin, one of the body's principal hormones. Insulin helps move blood sugar into cells where it should be burned for energy. However, insulin has far-reaching gene- and cell-regulating roles beyond that of glucose metabolism. For example, elevated insulin levels promote fat accumulation around the waist, stimulate hunger, and increase the risk of heart disease and cancer.

All of these changes result from insulin's altering the activity of a variety of genes. Insulin turns on genes that increase levels of the stress hormone cortisol, which accelerates aging. Insulin also increases the production of C-reactive protein, a substance that promotes inflammation and accelerates aging. One of the key steps you can take to minimize DNA and gene damage is to keep your insulin levels as low as possible. A fasting insulin of under 12 mcIU/ml of blood would be ideal, and some physicians recommend levels under 8 mcIU/ml. You can achieve this level by following the dietary recommendations in chapter 7.

Calorie Restriction: Reduced DNA Damage and Greater Longevity

Reducing your overall caloric intake, while maintaining adequate intake of vitamins and minerals, can reduce DNA damage, increase life expectancy, and lower the risk of disease. Animal studies dating back to

1935 have consistently shown that permanently cutting calorie intake by one-third extends the life expectancy of rodents by about 30 percent. However, experiments conducted in 2004 found that many of the benefits of lifetime calorie restriction may be achieved during late middle age.

Researchers long believed that this increase in life expectancy was the result of slowing down metabolism, and they were partly right. Scientists now understand that calorie-restricted diets also reduce the production of free radicals in mitochondria, largely because less food is broken down for energy. With fewer free radicals being formed, there is less opportunity for mitochondrial and nuclear DNA to become damaged.

Ongoing studies with monkeys, close biological relatives of humans, show that calorie restriction protects against many of the degenerative diseases typical of aging. Middle-aged calorie-restricted monkeys have lower blood sugar and insulin levels, look more youthful, exhibit higher energy levels, and show few signs of age-related degenerative diseases compared with animals that are allowed to eat as much as they want.

Granted, reducing caloric intake by one-third is not appealing for most people. However, nearly everyone can afford to eat somewhat smaller meals and resist the marketing of "supersized" meals that have resulted in overweight (supersized!) people. In addition, research suggests that some nutritional supplements, such as chromium picolinate and coenzyme Q10, may decrease cell damage in ways similar to calorie-restricted diets.

How Vitamins Reduced Barbara's Symptoms of Sickle-Cell Anemia

Barbara, age twenty-eight, was born with sickle-cell anemia, in which a genetic mutation interferes with the normal function of red blood cells and leads to their rapid breakdown. Her distant African ancestors benefited from this particular mutation, which conferred a measure of protection against the parasite causing malaria. But for Barbara, living in the malaria-free United States, the disease meant only chronic anemia, blood clots, episodes of pain, frequent colds, and most likely an early death from cardiovascular disease.

There is no way to fix or change the HbS mutation causing sickle-cell anemia. However, Barbara's physician had read recent medical journal reports showing that moderately high doses of some vitamin supplements could reduce the symptoms of sickle-cell anemia. He recommended that she take these supplements, including 800 IU of natural vitamin E, 4,000 mg of vitamin C, 1,000 mcg of folic acid, 500 mcg of vitamin B$_{12}$, and 4,000 mg of garlic supplements.

After several weeks Barbara's painful episodes began to decline. Six months later she reported having fewer episodes of pain and fewer colds, and tests indicated that her red blood cells were not breaking down as quickly as they had been. While the vitamins were not a cure for sickle-cell anemia, they did significantly minimize Barbara's symptoms.

Nutrient Deficiencies Inhibit Gene Activities

It is important to understand that inadequate levels of vitamins, minerals, and other types of micronutrients can impair normal gene function. Micronutrients play myriad roles in the body's production of new DNA, cells, and tissue, as well as in energy production.

For years many scientists and physicians dismissed the health benefits of vitamins and minerals. However, the importance of these micronutrients in synthesizing, protecting, and repairing DNA and genes is undeniable, if often buried in the technical language of biochemistry textbooks. Inadequate levels of vitamins and minerals become "rate-limiting" factors—that is, they slow or inhibit the rate of necessary chemical reactions.

If this idea seems a bit arcane, consider that the rates of these chemical reactions affect your heart function, your healing time, your energy levels, your thinking and memory, your resistance to infection and cancer, your body's ability to detoxify noxious chemicals, and every other physical function. Low levels and outright deficiencies of micronutrients slow and inhibit genetic activities and chemical reactions, resulting at first in vague symptoms and later in diagnosed diseases. Optimal levels of vitamins and other micronutrients promote the necessary genetic activities and chemical reactions of health.

How Poor Nutrition Affects Subsequent Generations

If nutritional deficiencies or imbalances can impair DNA function and set the stage for disastrous health consequences in an individual, what might be the effect of a genetically inadequate diet on that person's children and even grandchildren?

Many studies have investigated how nutritional excesses or deficiencies early in life affect a person in later years, as well as subsequent generations. They may permanently alter an individual's lifelong nutritional requirements, and genetic changes may be passed on to future family members.

As one example, the Canadian psychiatrist Dr. Abram Hoffer found that prisoners of war, who suffered severe nutritional deficiencies while in captivity, developed exaggerated requirements for many micronutrients, such as the B vitamins. These increased requirements for B vitamins suggest that the prisoners of war suffered a combination of genetic damage and permanent biochemical impairments. The consequences of nutritional deficiencies could be overcome through high-dose vitamin supplementation.

In addition, physicians have recognized that people who are obese or have diabetes are likely to have children who also develop these conditions. Such diseases in the children of obese or diabetic parents have often been vaguely attributed to either genetics or poor eating habits. While parents often share bad dietary habits with their children, there is strong evidence that some genetic changes in parents can be passed on to children and grandchildren.

A recent study published in the *European Journal of Human Genetics* confirmed the multigenerational effects of different eating habits in people. Swedish researchers tracked three generations of people, born in 1890, 1905, and 1920, and analyzed the effects of abundant dietary carbohydrates (during times of food surplus) and carbohydrate restriction (during times of famine) on subsequent generations.

The researchers found that if a person's father or paternal grandfather ate a lot of carbohydrates before puberty, his children and grandchildren had a higher risk of dying from cardiovascular disease and were four times more likely to develop diabetes. However, if a person's father or grandfather consumed fewer carbohydrates, his children and grandchildren were far less likely to develop either diabetes or cardiovascular disease. These differences in disease risk reflect fundamental alterations in gene behavior and biochemistry from one generation to the next.

In a similar vein, recent studies have shown that the diet of pregnant mice can significantly influence their offspring's appearance and risk of disease. Researchers at the Duke University Medical Center experimented with a breed of mice possessing a gene that codes for yellow fur, obesity, and a greater risk of diabetes. But when the researchers gave pregnant mice extra B-complex vitamins, the gene was turned off in the fetuses, so they grew up thin and with brown fur and had a lower long-term risk of disease. This study, and its implications in people, will be discussed further in chapter 5, while some of the implications of prenatal stresses and nutrition will be described in chapter 9.

How Extra Vitamin D Offset a Sluggish VDR Gene

After experiencing two falls and fractured bones, Sandy, age fifty-five, was diagnosed with osteoporosis. Her physician recommended that she take a daily supplement containing 1,000 mg of calcium and 400 IU of vitamin D. But the supplement did not seem to help. A year later she fractured her wrist while loading groceries into her car.

A new physician suggested that Sandy take part in a university-based study on genetics and osteoporosis. Tests revealed that Sandy had a common polymorphism (variation) in the vitamin D receptor gene (VDR), which regulates how the body uses vitamin D and calcium. Because of the VDR polymorphism, Sandy did not efficiently use vitamin D, and her blood levels of the vitamin remained low.

Her physician recommended three steps. He increased Sandy's vitamin D intake to 2,000 IU daily. He suggested that she spend fifteen to thirty minutes a day walking in the sun, which would help her body make its own vitamin D. He also recommended that Sandy begin some moderate weight training, because resistance exercise increases bone density.

Two years later bone scans have shown an increase in Sandy's bone density. In addition, despite her heightened level of activity, she has not experienced any additional fractures. Her higher supplemental intake of vitamin D, combined with regular sun exposure, has successfully overcome an inefficient VDR gene.

The Genetic Basis of Optimal Nutrition

If our ancient nutrient-dense diet established our genetic baseline, what guidelines might we follow for getting the most out of our genes today, especially when we are living longer and acquiring more age-related genetic damage?

After the discovery of vitamins in 1911, considerable medical attention focused on identifying and correcting the most severe nutritional deficiencies. These gross deficiencies—resulting in diseases like scurvy, pellagra, beri-beri, and others—were relatively common during the early part of the twentieth century. Providing vitamin-rich foods (and, later, vitamin supplements) corrected the symptoms of these deficiency diseases. However, nearly all researchers and physicians at the time made an incorrect assumption: they believed that the symptoms were the early signs of vitamin deficiencies. In truth, the deficiency diseases were actually the most serious and advanced symptoms of vitamin deficiencies, representing a near-total breakdown of normal gene function and biochemistry before death.

In 1939, which might seem like an eternity ago, Dr. Albert Szent-Györgyi, the Nobel laureate who discovered vitamin C, proposed that the medical community shift its focus from determining minimal or adequate vitamin levels to gauging the optimal levels of vitamins that people should consume. A growing number of nutritionally oriented physicians have done just this, using dietary changes and nutritional supplements to treat a wide variety of diseases.

As brief examples, many different diseases can be prevented or reversed through a variety of nutritional therapies. Among them are Alzheimer's disease (vitamin E), carpal tunnel syndrome (vitamin B_6), macular degeneration (lutein) migraine headache (vitamin B_2 or magnesium), mood disorders (B-complex vitamins), multiple sclerosis (vitamins D and B_{12}), night blindness (vitamin A), Parkinson's disease (coenzyme Q10), periodontal disease (vitamin C), and stroke (vitamin C). Underlying all of these diseases are damaged or malfunctioning genes, a consequence of consuming inadequate amounts of the nutritional precursors to DNA and various biochemicals.

It is important to remember that while we all require the same nutrients for health, we often need them in substantially different amounts. Research along these lines was first conducted by Roger J. Williams, Ph.D., in the 1950s. In other words, you may achieve reasonable good health by consuming about 200 mg of vitamin C daily, whereas I may need ten or more times that amount. The reasons relate to our underlying biochemical and genetic individuality.

In the next three chapters, we will explore how specific nutrients are involved in generating energy, creating new and replacement DNA, and protecting and repairing DNA.

PART II

Gene-Enhancing Nutritional Supplements

4

Nutrients That Enhance Energy and Prevent DNA Damage

To make new DNA, which is necessary for health, healing, and life itself, your cells must have the energy to drive the underlying biological construction processes. When large numbers of cells lack this energy, the deficiency negatively affects the production of DNA and the function of genes in different organs. You cannot feel a reduction in the energy-producing chemical reactions in individual cells, but you will notice some of their collective consequences in the form of fatigue, mental fuzziness, and increased risk of illness.

The Role of Energy in DNA

Through a series of biochemical reactions known as bioenergetics, mitochondria in cells break down simple food molecules, such as glucose and fat, and convert them to adenosine triphosphate (ATP). The health of your DNA is dependent on two crucial roles played by ATP.

First, ATP functions as the universal form of chemical energy in cells, acting somewhat like an electrical capacitor that stores and quickly releases energy to drive chemical reactions, including the activities of DNA and RNA. The importance of cellular energy cannot be overstated; it has been described as the "currency" of life or, if you prefer, our "life force." This chemical energy powers every cell in your body.

Second, ATP is also an essential ingredient in the structure of DNA, contributing a structure that biochemists call an adenine ring. After being created in mitochondria, ATP molecules migrate through each cell to form part of the structure of both mitochondrial DNA and nuclear DNA.

Significantly, low levels of ATP or low levels of the nutrients involved in ATP production reduce cell energy levels and prevent normal cellular and DNA activities. The more obvious symptoms may include fatigue, organ dysfunction, and premature aging.

This chapter focuses primarily on the most important vitamin-like "mitochondrial nutrients" involved in ATP production. As you read about these nutrients, remember that as long as your cells can produce large amounts of ATP, they will have the energy to function and remain capable of making healthy new DNA and replacement cells. When you eat foods or take supplements high in these nutrients, you will likely sense an improvement in your energy levels, an outward sign of more efficient bioenergetics.

Bioenergetics: Converting Food to Energy

Bioenergetics occurs in two connected series of chemical reactions. The first group of chemical reactions takes place within what is known as the Krebs cycle. This cycle is analogous to a water wheel that uses the energy of moving water to rotate the wheel. During the Krebs cycle, glucose (made from all sugars and carbohydrates) and fat are broken down and converted to increasingly energetic compounds. Much of the resulting energy is channeled into another biochemical pathway called oxidative phosphorylation. You can envision this pathway as something like a trough carrying fast-moving water from the water wheel. This energy eventually leads to the creation of ATP.

There is, however, a paradox in these energy-generating reactions. While bioenergetics is absolutely essential for life, it also generates nearly all of the destructive free radicals made within the body. Free radicals are a necessary part of the chemical reactions, because they transfer much of the energy through the many chemical reactions. Most of the free radicals are contained within these chemical reactions, but some do leak out, leading to mitochondrial damage and, little by little, less efficient energy production, leading to a kind of chain reaction:

As bioenergetics becomes less efficient, more free radicals manage to escape. As these free radicals continue to increase and spread out, they damage DNA. As damage to DNA accumulates, energy production becomes even less efficient, leading eventually to organ failure or death.

Boosting Your Body's Energy Production

The good news is that you can take steps to improve the efficiency of bioenergetics. All of the chemical reactions in bioenergetics are built on nutrients, also known as nutritional substrates. While glucose and fat provide the raw fuel for energy, their combustion depends on the presence of several key nutrients. For example, coenzyme A plays a crucial role in the Krebs cycle, and coenzyme A is built around a molecule of pantethene, a form of the B vitamin pantothenic acid. Coenzyme A also helps molecules attach to each other, and it is essential for the creation of DNA and RNA.

Increasing your intake of mitochondrial nutrients found in foods and supplements can significantly improve the efficiency of your bioenergetics. The benefits are more energy for your cells to do their jobs, increased (nonstimulant) energy for you in your day-to-day activities, less risk of certain diseases, and reduced free-radical damage to your DNA. The crucial nutrients are coenzyme Q10 (CoQ10), alpha-lipoic acid, carnitine and acetyl-L-carnitine, ribose, creatine, and some of the B vitamins. Again, as you read about the benefits of these nutrients, remember that they all enhance the production or utilization of ATP, which helps drive normal DNA activity.

Coenzyme Q10

CoQ10 has an exceptional pedigree: it was the basis of the 1972 Nobel Prize for Chemistry because of its key role in shuttling around the energy-carrying electrons involved in bioenergetics. Although people make small amounts of CoQ10 within their bodies, it is for all practical purposes a vitamin.

The greatest concentrations of CoQ10 are found in the most energy-dependent and metabolically active cells, including those that form the skeletal muscle (in your arms and legs), the heart, the brain, the liver, and the immune system. In the late 1960s, Japanese researchers discovered that CoQ10 was beneficial in treating cardiomyopathy and heart failure, diseases in which the heart muscle lacks the energy to pump blood. In the 1980s and 1990s, a small number of American and European physicians also began using CoQ10 to treat cardiomyopathy and heart failure.

CoQ10, the Muscle Vitamin

One of the best ways to appreciate the role of CoQ10 is through a particular group of relatively rare inherited diseases. As you read in chapter 2, mitochondrial myopathies are caused by specific genetic defects that interfere with normal bioenergetics. In people born with mitochondrial myopathies, portions of mitochondrial DNA are damaged or missing, which results in incomplete or incoherent instructions for making energy. CoQ10 and other mitochondrial nutrients have been used to successfully treat many patients with these diseases.

Comparable damage to mitochondrial DNA develops during normal aging in otherwise healthy people. Many leading scientists, including Bruce N. Ames, Ph.D., of the University of California at Berkeley and Anthony Linnane, Ph.D., of Australia's Centre for Molecular Biology and Medicine, believe that problems with mitochondrial bioenergetics lie at the very root of the aging process and DNA damage.

Like most other micronutrients, CoQ10 multitasks—that is, it performs multiple functions in the body. Its primary function is in bioenergetics, helping cells complete their energy-producing chemical reactions. Its secondary function is as an antioxidant, in which it protects cell membranes from free-radical damage. Other CoQ10 functions, which include reducing blood pressure and improving glucose tolerance, hint at its ability to influence gene behavior.

How Betty Got Her Heart Back

Betty, who lives in Dallas, was diagnosed at age fifty with dilated idiopathic cardiomyopathy, a deadly weakening of the heart muscle. Her heart was enlarged and weak, pumping only a fraction of the blood her body needed and leaving her a virtual invalid. "It took everything I had to go from the bedroom to the bathroom," she recalls.

For two years Betty's physician treated her with conventional heart drugs. In the early 1980s, he asked her to participate in a clinical trial with CoQ10. In the study, Betty began taking 100 mg of CoQ10 and, after about six months, noticed that she had higher energy levels. Tests indicated that her heart had become smaller and was pumping blood more efficiently.

More than twenty years later, Betty remains in reasonably good health. She currently takes 200 mg of CoQ10, sometimes increasing the dosage when she feels stressed. On a recent vacation to Chicago, she was able to walk extensively with friends without feeling unduly tired.

"I feel pretty good most of the time, and I do almost everything except the heaviest yard work by myself," she says. "I need this vitamin to live. If I stop taking it, my heart will deteriorate again, and I'll be dead in a year."

CoQ10 Improves Energy Levels

CoQ10's role in energy production may be best illustrated by its value in treating cardiomyopathy and heart failure, conditions that often warrant a heart transplant. For example, Drs. Peter Langsjoen, of Tyler, Texas, and Stephen Sinatra, of Manchester, Connecticut, are nutritionally oriented cardiologists who have consistently used CoQ10 supplements, typically 300 to 400 mg daily, to treat cardiomyopathy and heart failure in thousands of patients. On many occasions patients on a waiting list for heart-transplant surgery regained normal heart function after taking CoQ10 supplements and no longer required surgery. CoQ10 supplements improve bioenergetics and increase ATP levels, but it is also possible that higher ATP levels support the production of new DNA and healthy new heart cells.

The ability of CoQ10 to boost mitochondrial activity and energy levels has been demonstrated in a variety of other studies in healthy and ill people. In one small study, Dr. Langsjoen asked several generally healthy octogenarian patients to take CoQ10 supplements. All the patients reported improved energy levels, and one even gained enough energy to chop firewood, a pastime that advancing age had previously forced him to give up.

Still other clinical research shows that CoQ10 can benefit people with muscular dystrophy, a crippling disease. In two separate studies, researchers found that patients receiving modest dosages (100 mg) of CoQ10 supplements daily exhibited increased endurance and less fatigue after three months. In a medical journal article, researchers described the case of one particular patient, a lawyer, who had muscular dystrophy. He had been told by his neurologist to prepare himself mentally for being confined to a wheelchair within two years. However, the patient started taking CoQ10 supplements, and six years later he was still leading an active life, swimming, playing golf, and practicing law in a demanding practice. Comparable benefits have been reported in patients with postpolio syndrome, a type of muscle weakness that returns decades after a person recovers from polio.

CoQ10 and Cancer

CoQ10 also improves the activity of immune cells, enhancing their ability to attack cancer cells. Cancer patients are typically deficient in CoQ10, a condition that appears to increase their risk of posttreatment cancer recurrence.

Dr. Knud Lockwood, a surgeon in Copenhagen, had been treating breast cancers for more than thirty-five years when he began recommending CoQ10 to his patients. Lockwood found that high-dose CoQ10 supplements (390 mg daily) prompted remissions in recurrent breast cancers. He and his colleagues wrote that CoQ10 probably does not have any direct antitumor properties but rather improves the energetic activity of the body's anticancer immune cells.

CoQ10 and Genetic Diseases

In addition to helping people with mitochondrial myopathies, CoQ10 supplements can also benefit those with some other types of inherited diseases. Two such conditions are retinitis pigmentosa, a disease that leads to blindness, and hereditary ataxia, which affects movement of the arms and legs.

Retinitis pigmentosa is characterized by the steady degeneration of the rods and cones of the retina, minute eye structures needed for normal vision. In a very small but promising clinical study, researchers from Italy's University of Bologna found that CoQ10 supplements improved vision and reversed the progression of retinitis pigmentosa.

In other studies researchers used very high dosages (300 to 3,000 mg daily) to treat six patients with hereditary ataxia. According to an article in *Neurology*, all improved by an average of 25 percent over the course of a year, gaining strength, developing better coordination and balance, and suffering fewer seizures. Five of the patients who had been confined to wheelchairs regained the ability to walk with some assistance.

CoQ10 and Parkinson's Disease

Parkinson's disease, a neurological disorder characterized by decreasing production of the neurotransmitter dopamine, results in symptoms such as tremors, slowness of movement, and muscle rigidity. In its later stages, Parkinson's disease often includes an Alzheimer-like dementia. Treatment with the drug levodopa temporarily slows the progression of the disease, but it increases the likelihood of dementia.

To test the potential benefits of CoQ10, Dr. Clifford W. Shults of the University of California at San Diego directed a study of 80 Parkinson patients at ten different U.S. hospitals. The patients received either 300, 600, or 1,200 mg of CoQ10 or placebos daily for sixteen weeks. At the end of the study, all the patients taking CoQ10 had less severe symptoms than did those in the placebo group. Patients taking the highest dosage of CoQ10 benefited the most, and their symptoms were only about half as severe as those of the people in the placebo group. An analysis of cells taken from patients confirmed that CoQ10 increased the energy-producing activity of their mitochondria.

CoQ10 Supplements Reenergize José

José knew all about energy—or at least his lack of it. At the end of an average day, he would settle into his recliner, watch television, and then doze off for an hour or two. That changed when he started taking 30 mg of CoQ10 daily.

José, who lives in the San Francisco Bay area, is in his midfifties and says that CoQ10 supplements enabled him to regain the energy levels he had about fifteen years ago. "I'm able to go out and have some semblance of a life, even after a hard day at work," he says.

And it's not just that he has more physical energy. Before José began taking CoQ10 supplements, he found himself agonizing over the simplest decisions. New tasks at work became difficult to learn, and he dreaded new assignments. He was also increasingly forgetful, so much so that he thought he was suffering early signs of Alzheimer's disease.

"Since starting CoQ10, I'm much more able to concentrate, and learning is no more difficult than it was in my youth," he added. "I'm convinced that if CoQ10 is not life-extending, it is at the very least life-quality-enhancing for those who are deficient in it."

Statin Drugs Reduce CoQ10 Levels

Fatigue, liver disease, and heart failure are among the risks associated with "statin" drugs, the largest category of cholesterol-lowering drugs (which include Lipitor, Mevacor, Pravachol, Zocor, and the now banned Baycol). According to studies by Dr. Peter Langsjoen and many other researchers, statin drugs also decrease the body's production of CoQ10.

These drugs work by reducing the activity of a key enzyme involved in the production of cholesterol. However, the same enzyme is needed for CoQ10 synthesis. So with great irony, drugs prescribed to lower the risk of a heart attack increase the risk of fatigue and heart failure.

For the most part, the pharmaceutical companies do not publicize this side effect of statin drugs. Yet Merck, the maker of Zocor, owns two patents describing the combination of its statin drug and CoQ10. So anyone taking statin drugs should also take supplemental CoQ10.

How to Take CoQ10 Supplements

The striking results obtained from CoQ10 supplements may make this nutrient seem a little like a panacea. However, whenever nutrients positively affect bioenergetics and DNA, they will likely have diverse effects on health and well-being. Here are some supplement guidelines to follow:

- If you are under age forty and in good health, take 30 to 50 mg of CoQ10 daily.
- If you are over age forty and in good health, take 50 to 100 mg daily.
- If you have risk factors for any of the diseases discussed in this section, take 100 mg daily. This dosage is also appropriate for people taking statin drugs, and you do not have to adjust the amount of the statin.
- If you have cardiomyopathy, heart failure, or cancer, work with your physician to establish a dosage of 300 to 400 mg daily. If you take any kind of heart-stimulating medication, including but not limited to digitalis or beta-blockers, your medication requirements will likely decrease as CoQ10 naturally improves your heart function. Please work with your physician to adjust the dosage of the medication.

Alpha-Lipoic Acid

Another vitamin-like substance, alpha-lipoic acid, serves multiple functions in the energy-generating Krebs cycle. In addition to aiding the breakdown of food into energy, alpha-lipoic acid improves the efficiency of insulin, a hormone that regulates blood-sugar levels and some aspects of the aging process. Chronically elevated insulin levels (hyperinsulinemia), which occur in diabetes, prediabetes, and Syndrome X, lead to abnormal gene activity, accelerated aging, and higher risks of obesity, heart disease, and cancer. It is far healthier to maintain relatively low and efficient levels of insulin, and supplemental alpha-lipoic acid can help you accomplish this.

Like other micronutrients, alpha-lipoic acid serves a multitude of roles in maintaining and restoring health. It significantly increases chemical reactions in the liver that in turn speed the breakdown of toxins, including pollutants, and drugs. It boosts the body's production of glutathione compounds, the most powerful family of antioxidants made by the body. It also helps regenerate vitamins E and C and CoQ10 after they become chemically exhausted from fighting free radicals.

In addition, alpha-lipoic acid suppresses the activity of "nuclear factor kappa beta," a gene-transcription protein that turns on genes that promote inflammation, cancer, and replication of the human immunodeficiency virus. Chronic inflammation is involved in nearly all diseases, and so alpha-lipoic acid can reduce harmful gene activity.

Alpha-Lipoic Acid, Blood Sugar, and Insulin

Alpha-lipoic acid has been used (600 mg daily) for more than two decades in Germany to treat diabetic polyneuropathy, a degenerative nerve-disease complication of diabetes. The same dosage significantly improves the function of insulin and lowers insulin levels, a change that is often accompanied with a reduction in blood-sugar levels.

In addition to improving insulin function, supplemental alpha-lipoic acid leads to increases in ATP. This role was clearly shown in the description of a thirty-three-year-old woman treated by physicians at the University of Bologna. As a child the woman had been thin, weak, and intolerant of exercise. By her early twenties, she had developed eye-muscle disorders and droopy eyelids, a common sign of mitochondrial myopathies. On examination in her early thirties, she had very weak arm and leg muscles. A biopsy and other tests found that her body's cells were producing low levels of ATP. The woman's treatment consisted of 200 mg of alpha-lipoic acid three times daily. After several months new tests indicated that her ATP production had increased substantially and her symptoms had improved as well.

Alpha-Lipoic Acid, Mitochondria, and Age Reversal

Recently Bruce N. Ames, Ph.D., of the University of California at Berkeley and Tory Hagen, Ph.D., of Oregon State University conducted a series of animal experiments to explore the combined benefits of alpha-lipoic acid and another nutrient, acetyl-L-carnitine, on mitochondrial energy production and several signs of aging. (Carnitine and acetyl-L-carnitine will be discussed in the next section.) Although the experiments were conducted on laboratory rats, the results have important implications for people.

In one phase of the experiments, Ames and Hagen fed alpha-lipoic acid and acetyl-L-carnitine to groups of old and young rats. Old rats are typically lethargic and have only about one-third the energy of young rats. After several weeks of supplementation, the two nutrients had a dramatic rejuvenating and energy-boosting effect. The old rats' physical activity doubled and was almost identical to that of nonsupplemented young rats. The improvements, according to the researchers, were like taking a seventy-five-year-old woman and restoring her to the vigor of someone half her age. Ames and Hagen also reported comparable improvements in the animals' memories.

How to Take Alpha-Lipoic Acid Supplements

Alpha-lipoic acid is abundant in meat and broccoli, but only supplements can provide higher and clearly beneficial levels. Here are some supplement guidelines to follow:

- If you are in good health and plan to take alpha-lipoic acid as a general antioxidant or in combination with other supplements discussed in this chapter, take 50 to 100 mg daily.
- If you have diabetes, take the typical dosage used in Europe—200 mg three times daily—but do so under the guidance of a physician, since alpha-lipoic acid will probably decrease your requirements for glucose-regulating drugs, such as glucophage and insulin.
- For prediabetes, insulin resistance, or Syndrome X, take 200 mg once or twice daily to improve insulin function and glucose metabolism. For additional guidelines in blood-sugar disorders, see my book *Syndrome X: The Complete Nutritional Program to Prevent and Reverse Insulin Resistance.*

Alpha-lipoic acid, like any other supplement, will work best when combined with a healthy overall diet. Specifically, a nutrient-dense diet, rich in lean, high-quality protein (fish and chicken) and vegetables will help moderate spikes in blood sugar and insulin. For additional dietary guidelines, see chapters 7 and 8.

Carnitine and Acetyl-L-Carnitine

Carnitine and acetyl-L-carnitine are two forms of the same vitamin-like substance, which is naturally concentrated in meat, particularly organ meats. Carnitine, in various chemical forms, helps transport fats into the Krebs cycle, where they are broken down for energy. Without adequate dietary or supplemental carnitine, fats are not efficiently burned for energy. Carnitine enhances the benefits of both CoQ10 and alpha-lipoic acid in energy production.

Carnitine and Fatigue

In one of the best demonstrations of carnitine's energy-boosting effect, Dr. Audius V. Plioplys and his colleagues at Mercy Hospital and Medical Center in Chicago treated 28 men and women diagnosed with chronic fatigue syndrome (CFS). The patients were given either 3 grams daily of carnitine or the prescription drug amantadine (sometimes prescribed for pain reduction in neurological diseases) for eight weeks, after which time the treatments were reversed for another eight weeks.

The differences between carnitine and the drug were striking. Patients taking carnitine improved in all eighteen of the clinical tests used to assess CFS, and the improvements were significant in twelve of the tests. Only 1 patient stopped taking carnitine because of gastrointestinal upset. In contrast, only 15 of the patients were able to tolerate amantadine for a full eight weeks, and none experienced any improvement in symptoms.

Supplements Create a Newfound Sense of Vitality

Sharon, age thirty-eight, knew all about energy—or rather her lack of it. Each weekday morning she'd drag herself and her two small children out of bed, push them off to school, and drive the "commute from hell" to her office. Nine hours later she'd do it all in reverse.

Back at home by 6:30 P.M., Sharon would feed and bathe her children, get them into bed, and do a load or two of laundry. Ready to relax and read a book as the clock inched toward 11:00

P.M., she would see that her evening had again slipped away. Sharon had wanted to do more and wished she had the energy to do more. She would collapse into bed wondering how she'd get up the next morning and do it all over again.

Sharon's life changed after being treated by Dr. Richard Kunin of San Francisco. A dietary survey and blood tests indicated that Sharon wasn't either consuming or using some of the nutrients essential to energy production. After she adopted a protein-rich diet and started taking supplements of carnitine and CoQ10, Sharon's energy levels perked up. She discovered a new vitality—feeling better than she had in years—and was now able to juggle the many stresses of her life.

The Carnitine-Vitamin C-Energy Connection

Researchers have long known that fatigue is a symptom of scurvy, the most severe stage of vitamin C deficiency, preceding death. But a study by Dr. Mark Levine of the National Institutes of Health found that the first two symptoms of short-term vitamin C deprivation (without scurvy) were fatigue and irritability, two symptoms common among North Americans.

Vitamin C is needed for the body's own production of carnitine, and low levels of the vitamin ultimately interfere with the burning of fats for energy. Carol Johnston, Ph.D., a professor of nutrition at Arizona State University, has pointed out that vitamin C supplements led to a 15 percent increase in endurance among athletes, a sign of improved bioenergetics. In addition, a 1984 study in the journal *Nutrition and Health* suggested that vitamin C (and, by implication, other mitochondrial nutrients) might even help promote weight loss.

How to Take Carnitine Supplements

Carnitine supplements are best consumed with a protein-rich meal, such as an omelette for breakfast or chicken, fish, or meat for dinner. Here are some supplement guidelines to follow:

- If you are generally healthy but feel a need to increase your energy levels, take 500 to 1,000 mg of carnitine daily.
- If you regularly feel fatigued, take 2,000 mg of carnitine with a high-protein, low-carbohydrate dinner. There is a good chance you will wake up the next morning feeling more energized. Continue daily supplementation.

- If you suffer from chronic fatigue syndrome, take 3,000 mg of carnitine daily. It may be helpful to take also 100 mg of CoQ10 and 100 mg of alpha-lipoic acid.

The acetyl-L-carnitine form of this nutrient seems to have more of an age-reversing effect, particularly on cognition and recall. However, it is considerably more expensive than regular carnitine. If you have serious problems with concentration or memory, the acetyl-L-carnitine form may be preferable to carnitine.

Ribose

Ribose forms the carbohydrate backbone of DNA and RNA, as well as that of vitamins B_2 and B_{12}. It is also one of the building blocks of ATP, the body's principal energy-containing molecule, and research suggests that ribose supplements can help maintain ATP levels.

Many runners, triathletes, and bodybuilders take ribose supplements to boost their stamina and strength. By doing so they increase their mitochondrial activity and fuel reserves for their cells. A study of male bodybuilders at the University of Nebraska found that taking supplemental ribose (10 grams daily) for several weeks led to increases in stamina and bench-press strength, compared with those in men taking placebos.

Ribose and Energy Production

Considerable research also indicates that ribose supplements can improve heart function in patients with congestive heart failure, as well as reduce pain and stiffness in overused muscles. All these benefits can be traced to improved bioenergetics and the replenishment of ATP. Significant quantities of ATP are often lost from heart and muscle cells that are overworked or do not receive enough blood to supply increased oxygen demands. In fact, your body uses ATP in amounts equal (through recycling) to your total body weight each day.

To make and recycle ATP, your cells need adequate amounts of chemicals called adenine nucleotides, the existence of which ultimately depends on the presence of ribose. Although ribose is produced in all cells, low levels of its building blocks in heart and muscle cells can limit production. Supplements sidestep the body's production of ribose and make it available quickly for heart and muscle cells.

Ribose and the Heart

In a recent study published in the *European Journal of Heart Failure*, Dr. Heyder Omran, a cardiologist at the University of Bonn, used ribose to treat 15 patients with coronary artery disease and congestive heart failure. The patients took either 5 grams of ribose or a placebo three times daily for three weeks. The supplements were then switched for another three-week period, so each patient took both ribose and the placebo at some point during the study. Patients developed more efficient heart-pumping action when taking ribose. The supplement also improved exercise stamina and overall quality of life. No improvements occurred when patients took placebos.

How to Take Ribose Supplements

If you are already taking CoQ10, alpha-lipoic acid, and carnitine, adding ribose may lead to an incremental (rather than significant) increase in energy.

- For improved energy levels, take 1,000 to 2,000 mg of ribose daily.
- If you regularly engage in strenuous exercise, consider taking up to 5 grams of ribose before exercising and 5 grams immediately afterward, during your cooldown phase.
- If you have heart disease, you might benefit from 5 grams of ribose two or three times daily. However, take it under the guidance of a physician, because your requirements for heart medications may decrease.

Creatine

Just as they did with ribose supplements, bodybuilders pioneered the use of creatine supplements for increasing strength, endurance, and muscle mass. Creatine helps the body recycle used ATP back to full strength. After ATP releases energy, it turns into adenosine diphosphate (ADP). Creatine helps ADP rapidly convert back to ATP. Considerable research supports its use in boosting bioenergetics on the cellular level and athletics and heart function on more obvious levels.

Creatine and Genetic Disorders

A study by Dr. Mark Tanopolsky of the McMaster University Medical School in Hamilton, Ontario, tested the effects of creatine supplements on 102 patients with muscular dystrophies, mitochondrial myopathies, and other disorders affecting bioenergetics. The patients were given 10 grams of creatine daily for five days, followed by 5 grams daily for an average of six days. People receiving the creatine had significant improvements in strength, enabling them to better perform high-intensity exercises.

Creatine might also prove helpful in the treatment of amyotrophic lateral sclerosis (ALS), known also as Lou Gehrig's disease. Dr. M. Flint Beal of the Harvard Medical School fed either normal or creatine-supplemented diets to mice bred to develop ALS. During the course of the experiment, nonsupplemented mice had 49 to 95 percent declines in the number of their brain cells. Meanwhile, animals receiving creatine maintained better physical motor activity and lived longer than the nonsupplemented mice. In the same experiment, creatine also outperformed the drug riluzole. Mice receiving a diet containing 2 percent creatine lived thirteen days longer than mice receiving riluzole and twenty-six days longer than the untreated animals.

How to Take Creatine Supplements

Start creatine supplementation by taking a "loading" dose of 10 grams daily for one week to saturate tissues. After the first week, decrease the dosage to 5 grams daily.

B-Complex Vitamins and NADH

Several B-complex vitamins play central roles in the Krebs cycle, literally functioning as the hub for all the other nutritional spokes. In particular, vitamins B_2 (riboflavin) and B_3 (niacinamide) sit at the center of energy production, enabling cells to perform various tasks, including the making of new DNA.

Patients with chronic fatigue syndrome are commonly deficient in B vitamins, a factor in their poor bioenergetics and low energy levels. High-potency B-complex vitamins (along with vitamin C to enhance carnitine synthesis) are often helpful.

Another supplement, NADH, which is built around vitamin B_3, has also been shown helpful in fatigue. Dr. Joseph A. Bellanti and colleagues at Georgetown University in Washington, D.C., treated 26 patients suffering from chronic fatigue syndrome with 10 mg of vitamin NADH or a placebo daily for four weeks. After the four-week "washout period," the NADH and placebo treatments were reversed. Eight (31 percent) of the 26 patients responded to NADH supplements with about a 10 percent reduction in chronic fatigue symptoms. In contrast, only 2 subjects (8 percent) responded favorably to the placebo.

How to Take B Vitamins and NADH Supplements

If you take a multivitamin supplement, you are already getting B-complex vitamins. However, the dosage in many brands is too low to be of much benefit.

- For general health maintenance, be sure your multivitamin or B-complex supplement contains at least 10 mg of vitamin B_1, 10 mg of vitamin B_2, and 10 mg of B_3.
- If you feel anxious, stressed, or depressed, take a B-complex vitamin supplement that contains 50 to 100 mg each of vitamins B_1, B_2, and B_3. In general, the other B vitamins in the formula will be in appropriate ratios.
- If you regularly feel fatigued, take a B-complex supplement with 100 mg each of vitamin B_1, B_2, and B_3, plus 10 mg of NADH.

Physical Activity and Gene Activity

While these nutrients are essential for your body's normal production of energy, physical activity also plays a crucial role. Exercise increases the burning of calories, reduces fat, and increases muscle—all of which improve utilization of various mitochondrial nutrients.

In an article in the July/August 2004 issue of *Nutrition*, researchers from the University of Texas presented a brief overview of how exercise turns some genes on and others off. These changes in gene activity underlie the more obvious physiological changes related to endurance, fat loss, and muscle gain. For example, exercise turns on the FAT/CD36 gene, which increases the burning of fats. It also enhances activity of the PDH gene, which regulates the burning of carbohydrates. In addition, exercise boosts activity of the ADRB2 gene, which promotes the burning of fat from the body's fat cells.

In the next chapter, we will look at how B vitamins and other nutrients are involved in the creation of new molecules, particularly those involved in making, repairing, and regulating DNA.

5

Nutrients That Make and Repair DNA

Whenever a cell in your body makes a copy of itself, which is necessary for normal growth, repair of injuries, and replacement of damaged or old cells, it must first duplicate all 3 billion of the chemical letters forming its DNA. The DNA copy is earmarked for the new cell, and it will direct the functions of that new cell.

Inevitably, the quality of your DNA deteriorates slightly during normal cell replication, leading to errors in the new cell's biological instructions. It's like taking a photograph of a photograph; the copy will never be quite as good as the original. The mistakes made during normal DNA replication, as well as ongoing free-radical damage, lead to age-related changes in cells and an increased risk of malfunctioning, which eventually manifests as disease.

However, it is possible to enhance the accuracy of your DNA replication and repair processes through a good diet and the use of certain nutritional supplements. Although healthy foods provide the foundation of healthy DNA, supplemental nutrients (in capsules or tablets) help ensure that adequate amounts of the DNA building blocks are present in cells.

Two families of nutrients play critical roles in this regard. First, several B-complex vitamins are vital to the synthesis, repair, and regulation of DNA. Second, amino acids, which make up the protein you eat, are needed by DNA to make your own body's proteins, enzymes, and hormones. The first part of this chapter will focus on DNA synthesis, repair, and regulation, and the second part will describe the role of amino acids.

Vitamins as the Building Blocks of Your DNA

Despite the billions of dollars that have been spent on gene research, most scientists have ignored the fundamental dependence of DNA on B-complex vitamins. Indeed, much of the science of B vitamins and DNA synthesis and repair is mentioned only briefly in biochemistry books.

Key B Vitamins for DNA Synthesis

Your body needs several B vitamins to make DNA nucleotide bases, the molecules that form the chemical letters—adenine, cytosine, guanine, and thymine—of the DNA alphabet. In the simplest terms, thymine synthesis requires vitamins B_3 and B_6 and folic acid; cytosine needs vitamin B_3; and guanine and adenine require vitamin B_3 and folic acid. Without these vitamins, DNA would not exist—that is why they are cofactors to normal DNA synthesis, repair, and function.

These B-complex vitamins support what biochemists refer to as "one-carbon metabolism." Carbon, as you probably learned in school, forms the basis of all life on earth, and its role in DNA synthesis is but one example of its essential role in your life and health. In addition to supporting DNA synthesis, these vitamins have many other roles in maintaining physical and mental health.

Folic Acid. While several B vitamins donate carbon atoms to the biochemical reactions involved in DNA synthesis, folic acid may be the most crucial. It both donates and accepts (for transfer to additional chemical reactions) one-carbon atoms, while varying chemical forms of folic acid foster a variety of biochemical reactions. For example, one form of folic acid is required for the synthesis of DNA, while a slightly different form works with vitamin B_{12} to build more complex molecules throughout the body. In addition, a specific type of chemical reaction, called DNA methylation (to be discussed shortly) influences the behavior of DNA with far-reaching consequences.

Vitamin B_{12}. Cells require vitamin B_{12} during the synthesis of new DNA, as well as for the molecule-building process of methylation. Studies by Michael Fenech, Ph.D., a researcher at Australia's Commonwealth Scientific and Industrial Research Organization, have found that both young and elderly men with low blood levels of vitamin B_{12} and folic acid suffer a high rate of serious DNA damage. Such damage accelerates the aging of cells and also increases the risk of developing cancer.

Vitamin B_6. Known also as pyridoxine, vitamin B_6 is converted by cells to pyridoxal 5'-phosphate, the biologically active form of this nutrient. (Pyridoxal 5'-phosphate is available in supplement form, but it is more expensive than regular vitamin B_6.) Vitamin B_6 is needed for the production of serine hydroxymethylase, an enzyme involved in one-carbon metabolism and in the synthesis of DNA.

Vitamin B_3. Known as niacin (nicotinic acid) and niacinamide (nicotinamide), vitamin B_3 plays a central role in the production of energy and ATP. As discussed in chapter 4, some ATP is incorporated into the structure of DNA.

Vitamin B_3 is also required for the cellular production of a key DNA repair enzyme, poly(ADP-ribose) polymerase. This enzyme, known simply as PARP, is literally built around vitamin B_3. Without sufficient vitamin B_3 to make PARP, cells cannot repair DNA damage from cancer-causing chemicals, and thus the risk of cancer is increased. Supplemental vitamin B3 helps reinforce DNA, especially when it is exposed to cancer-causing chemicals.

How B-Vitamin Deficiencies Affect DNA Repair

Many people are fearful of radiation exposure from nuclear power plants and other sources. However, according to Bruce N. Ames, Ph.D., one of the world's leading cell biologists and professor emeritus at the University of California at Berkeley, DNA damage from B-vitamin deficiencies is identical to damage caused by radiation. In both cases strands of DNA break apart. No reasonable person would unnecessarily expose himself to radiation, so why would anyone want to suffer the same damage from low intake of B vitamins?

Unfortunately, up to 10 percent of Americans are deficient in at least one B vitamin, based on very conservative governmental recommendations for intake. In actuality, the number of Americans with either marginal intake or one or more B-vitamin deficiencies is likely several times higher. Low intake of any one of the B vitamins will slow or inhibit the synthesis of new DNA and its repair.

Specifically, low levels of vitamin B_3 lead to genetic instability, chromosome fragility, and breaks in DNA strands. Studies have found that low levels of vitamin B_2, which plays a role in DNA repair enzymes, also lead to more breaks in DNA. Similarly, low intake of vitamin B_6 inhibits the effectiveness of enzymes involved in DNA synthesis.

People with marginal intake of folic acid also have a high rate of chromosome damage, which can be corrected with supplementation. Folic acid deficiency during the early weeks of pregnancy can impair DNA synthesis in the rapidly growing fetus and cause a variety of birth defects, including spina bifida, cleft palate, and cleft lip.

How exactly does folic acid deficiency lead to DNA damage? When people are deficient in folic acid, cells cannot synthesize adequate amounts of thymine, one of the chemical letters of DNA. Instead DNA incorporates large amounts of uracil, which is normally used only to make RNA. But uracil has no function in DNA, and so DNA repair enzymes remove the uracil, which leaves breaks in the DNA. These breaks are like missing links in a chain, and they wreak havoc on a cell's genetic programming. With the restoration of adequate levels of folic acid to the diet, thymine is properly incorporated into DNA. Low levels of vitamins B_6 and B_{12} also interfere with thymine production, with an effect similar to that of folic acid deficiency.

On a daily basis, you cannot feel a decrease in normal DNA synthesis. However, you can see the end result. People who are slow to heal from cuts and scrapes are often deficient in these and other nutrients, and slow healing is just one sign of sluggish DNA synthesis. Long-term poor DNA synthesis and higher levels of uncorrected DNA damage set the stage for cancer, heart disease, Alzheimer's disease, birth defects, and miscarriage. Some research even indicates that low levels of folic acid can interfere with normal brain development.

Vitamins Help Crystal Have a Healthy Baby

Crystal, age thirty-three, had experienced more than her share of difficulties on the road to motherhood. During her twenties she miscarried once, gave birth to a stillborn baby, and delivered a son with spina bifida, a serious birth defect that led to his death several months later.

A new physician, looking at Crystal's medical history, recommended that she undergo genetic testing for a subtle defect in the gene coding for methylenetetrahydrofolate reductase (MTHFR). MTHFR is an enzyme needed for the normal utilization of folic acid, and both the genetic defect and low folic acid intake have been associated with a higher risk of birth defects.

It turned out that Crystal did have that genetic defect, and a simple blood test also revealed that she had elevated levels of homocysteine, a sign of inadequate folic acid intake. Following her physician's recommendation, Crystal began eating more spinach and dark green lettuces, good sources of folic acid, and taking a B-complex supplement plus 1,000 mcg of extra folic acid. Her doctor also recommended that she eat fewer sweets, because diets high in sugar have also been linked to a greater risk of birth defects.

Last year Crystal gave birth to a healthy eight-pound girl, and she and her husband are planning to have another baby in the next couple of years. Crystal's improved eating habits and the B-vitamin supplements she now takes successfully counteracted an inborn genetic weakness.

How B Vitamins Regulate Gene Function

The behavior of your genes is also influenced by methylation reactions and the presence of "methyl groups." These methyl groups, which are molecules containing three hydrogen atoms and one carbon atom, attach to DNA under a variety of circumstances and influence the expression, or activity, of genes.

DNA methylation most often serves to shut down specific genes when they are not needed, according to Craig A. Cooney, Ph.D., an assistant professor and expert on methylation at the University of Arkansas for Medical Sciences. Without DNA methylation, genes would operate with no restraint. For example, genes involved in liver function would become active in heart cells, leading to a cacophony of unwanted gene activity. (Each cell contains a full suite of DNA, so it is important that not all genes be operating simultaneously.) Thus DNA methylation helps regulate the normal behavior of DNA, much the way a traffic light regulates the flow of traffic.

This control of DNA activity through methylation becomes dysfunctional in cancer cells, which grow in an uncontrollable fashion. Cancer-causing genes, called oncogenes, turn on when they are not suppressed through methylation. Meanwhile, established cancers usually have an abnormally low rate of methylation. In the chaos of cancer, a lack of folic acid leads to poor suppression of oncogenes and damage to the p53 gene, changes that prevent this gene from performing its cancer-suppressing job.

Recent research has shown that supplemental B vitamins can

sometimes permanently alter DNA methylation patterns and in the process change what scientists have believed to be fixed genetic traits, such as physical appearance.

In separate experiments two teams of researchers worked with mice having a strong genetic propensity for yellow fur, obesity, diabetes, and heart disease, characteristics that have been traced back to the activity of the animals' "agouti" gene. Because of the agouti gene, these mice usually give birth to offspring that have yellow fur, are likely to become obese, and suffer a high risk of diabetes (related in part to obesity) and cancer. But when the researchers fed pregnant mice extra folic acid, vitamin B_{12}, choline, and betaine (all nutrients involved in methylation reactions), their offspring were thin, had brown fur, and had a low risk of disease.

Although the scientists involved in these experiments were reluctant to extend their animal findings to humans, they did demonstrate the powerful—and previously unknown—effect nutrients have on gene activity, without altering or mutating the structure of the gene. The implications in the field of genetics are profound: it is conceivable that any number of nutrients are capable of altering genetically "fixed" traits during fetal development. These particular studies also suggest that the current epidemic of obesity—two-thirds of Americans are overweight or obese—might be related to low intake of B vitamins (and poor methylation reactions), as well as to excess consumption of carbohydrate and fat calories.

How Vitamins Prevented Schizophrenia

An estimated 1 percent of people have a genetic predisposition for schizophrenia, which may be triggered by extreme psychological stress. The child of one schizophrenic parent has a 10 percent chance of developing the disease, characterized by hallucinations and delusions, and the child of two schizophrenic parents has a 50 percent chance of developing the disease.

Robert was diagnosed with schizophrenia and referred for treatment to Dr. Abram Hoffer, a Canadian psychiatrist. Hoffer, one of the pioneers in the medical use of vitamins, treated Robert with 3,000 mg of niacin (a form of vitamin B_3) and 3,000 mg of vitamin C daily. Robert recovered, became gainfully employed, married, and fathered four children. Several years later another psychiatrist told Robert that the vitamins were of no value, so he stopped taking them. His psychotic behavior returned and became so annoying to the community that he was asked to leave or to be committed to a mental hospital.

Robert and his wife, who was also schizophrenic, eventually sought treatment from Hoffer. Both recovered and went on to have satisfying careers. Three of their children excreted krypto-pyrrole (see "Pyroluria" in chapter 10), indicating that they were genetically at risk for one type of schizophrenia. The children were also placed on a vitamin regimen, and they have remained well for years.

Hoffer has pointed out that schizophrenics often end up being welfare recipients. He judges successful treatment at least in part based on whether people with schizophrenia are able to return to work and pay income taxes. "The treatment for this family repre-sents what nutritional therapy is all about," he says.

Note: the niacin (but not niacinamide) form of vitamin B_3 results in a strong tingling and flushing sensation that lasts for about an hour.

Methylation Reactions and Molecule-Building Processes

Other types of methylation reactions, which similarly depend on folic acid, vitamins B_6 and B_{12}, and several other nutrients, affect many other biochemical processes in the body. These methylation reactions con-tribute groups of hydrogen and carbon atoms to myriad biochemical reactions, influencing the body's production of neurotransmitters (affecting behavior), phospholipids (influencing the nervous system and levels of blood fats), and the synthesis of many other tissues (such as cartilage in knee joints). When these methylation reactions are faulty, they also increase the risk of DNA damage and the resultant diseases.

When methylation reactions become sluggish, all of the subsequent molecule- and cell-building reactions begin to stall. One sign of sluggish or defective methylation is an elevation in the blood levels of homo-cysteine. Homocysteine is highly toxic and damages blood-vessel walls, leading to the subsequent deposition of cholesterol, the body's attempt to deal with this damage.

Elevated homocysteine levels were first proposed as a risk factor for coronary heart disease by Dr. Kilmer McCully in 1969, at a time when medicine was committed to the idea that excess cholesterol was a leading cause of heart disease. Since the early 1990s, hundreds of studies have confirmed homocysteine as a leading risk factor for heart disease, stroke, Alzheimer's disease, and many other diseases.

Today many physicians routinely measure their patients' levels of homocysteine to assess their risk of heart disease. (Ideal homocysteine levels are less than 6 micromoles per liter of blood, and levels above 13 micromoles per liter are a serious risk factor.) No drug will lower homocysteine levels; only folic acid, vitamins B_6 and B_{12}, choline, and betaine can. But despite considerable attention to homocysteine in the medical journals, most physicians see it only as a risk factor for heart disease, not as a sign of seriously impaired methylation and chemical reactions throughout the body. Furthermore, excess homocysteine is also toxic to the methylation process and to many different types of cells in the body, likely damaging brain cells and creating mutations that give rise to some cancer cells.

Some population groups, ranging from about 7 percent of Irish to perhaps as much as 42 percent of French Canadians, carry a subtle genetic defect (technically known as a polymorphism) that reduces their bodies' ability to use folic acid efficiently. This genetic polymorphism produces an inefficient form of methylenetetrahydrofolate reductase (MTHFR), a key enzyme involved in using folic acid. Either a diet high in folic acid (found in dark leafy green vegetables) or folic acid supplements can offset this polymorphism, improve methylation, and lower homocysteine levels. The effect is comparable to "loading," or saturating, MTHFR's cellular environment with folic acid to improve its activity.

The many articles on homocysteine and folic acid in medical journals indicate that large numbers of people suffer from defective methylation, the result of inadequate intake of B vitamins. Some skeptical physicians have argued that while homocysteine is a risk factor for heart disease, no research shows that folic acid (or any other methyl nutrient) actually prevents heart disease. But over the past several years, some striking clinical studies have indeed found that folic acid supplements do lower the risk of heart disease, as well as the risk of serious complications after heart surgery. The beneficial effects of folic acid and other B vitamins on heart disease, birth defects, and so many other conditions point to their fundamental roles in maintaining healthy DNA and normal biochemistry.

Diseases associated with folic acid deficiency and poor methylation include the following:

CARDIOVASCULAR DISEASES

congestive heart failure   hypertension
coronary artery disease   stroke
hardening of the arteries

NEUROLOGICAL DISORDERS

Alzheimer's disease   depression
cognitive dysfunction   Parkinson's disease
  (perception, memory)

BIRTH DEFECTS

cleft lip   neural-tube defects (spina bifida)
cleft palate   spontaneous abortion
Down syndrome   (miscarriage)
infertility (male)

CANCERS

acute lymphocytic leukemia   colon cancer
breast cancer   stomach cancer
cervical cancer

Amino Acids and DNA

Amino acids form the chemical building blocks of protein, enzymes, and many hormones. When you eat a protein-containing food, such as chicken, the protein is broken down during digestion into its constituent amino acids. These amino acids are then delivered to cells, where DNA and RNA use them to construct more than fifty thousand new proteins for use in chemical reactions and in various tissue matrices of the body. For example, bone is not pure calcium but rather a matrix of highly specialized proteins along with calcium, magnesium, phosphorus, and other minerals.

Unfortunately, there are some confusing definitions of what are and are not "essential" dietary amino acids. Twenty dietary amino acids provide the basic components of all proteins and amino acids in the body. Nine of these amino acids are considered essential nutrients, because they *must* be obtained from the diet. Meanwhile, eleven other amino acids are considered nonessential, because the body can make them from the original nine. Unfortunately, the word "nonessential" conveys the impression that these amino acids are nutritionally unimportant.

The truth is that all twenty of these amino acids are required for health, and there are serious questions as to whether everyone, young and old, can efficiently make the eleven amino acids from the first nine. Animal foods are the most reliable sources of all of them. Vegetarian foods, like beans and nuts, provide "incomplete" proteins, in that they lack one or more of the essential amino acids. For this reason vegetarians must eat complementary proteins, such as those in legumes and brown rice, so they obtain all nine essential amino acids and some (or all) of the so-called nonessential ones. Vegetarians must be particularly conscientious about complementing their proteins, because incomplete proteins may be metabolized as carbohydrates rather than as true proteins.

To make a protein, DNA transfers an imprint of its instructions for that protein to RNA, which then uses amino acids in the cell to "cast" the protein, much the way a sculptor might use a plaster model to make a bronze figure. However, if all of the necessary amino acids are not present, the protein will not be produced, even if the DNA and RNA had the correct instructions. The inability of DNA to fully execute its instructions can impair any number of subsequent chemical reactions.

In some cases a DNA mutation codes for the incorrect amino acid, leading to disease. For example, sickle-cell anemia, an inherited disease characterized by crescent-shaped red blood cells instead of the normal round ones, results from a genetic mutation that uses an incorrect amino acid. This simple change alters the dynamics of red blood cells and makes them more likely to clot when they shouldn't.

The quality of amino acids available to DNA and RNA is influenced by our eating and cooking habits. Eating sugary foods and overcooking meat can create high levels of "advanced glycation end products," also known as AGEs, which essentially render proteins useless. AGEs form when proteins and sugars combine in a particular and undesirable way. They are especially nasty compounds, because they can attach to and damage DNA.

From the standpoint of minimizing AGE production, it is healthier to eat raw protein, and many people do eat raw fish in the form of sashimi. Raw meats are far more problematic because of the risk of bacterial and parasitic contamination, particularly with ground beef and chicken. One reasonable compromise is to lightly stir-fry food, which preserves quality protein while destroying harmful bacteria.

Some companies sell amino acid supplements, and nutritionally oriented physicians sometimes recommend individual or multiple amino acids to treat specific conditions. For example, arginine may be helpful in erectile dysfunction (it works the same way as Viagra), and the N-acetylcysteine form of cysteine can reduce cold and flu symptoms.

How to Take DNA-Building Nutrients

As a family of related nutrients, the B vitamins are so important to health that everyone should supplement with them.

- At the very least, for general health maintenance, take either a multivitamin or a B-complex supplement containing at least 10 mg of vitamin B_1, 10 mg of vitamin B_2, 10 mg of B_3, 400 mcg of folic acid, and 100 mcg of vitamin B_{12}.
- If you feel anxious, stressed, or depressed, take a B-complex vitamin supplement that contains 50 to 100 mg each of vitamins B_1, B_2, and B_3. In general, the other B vitamins in the formula will be in appropriate ratios.
- To limit gene damage, consider adding an additional 400 to 800 mcg of folic acid and 500 mcg of vitamin B_{12}.
- If you have had serious episodes of mental illness, such as severe depression or schizophrenia, you may benefit from still-higher dosages of individual B vitamins. Under these circumstances it might be best to consult with a nutritionally oriented physician or psychiatrist. For referrals go to www.orthomed.org or www.acam.org.

Please note that high dosages of vitamin B_2 will turn your urine bright yellow, but this is not harmful.

In the next chapter, we will focus on antioxidant nutrients, which help protect DNA from damage and also turn some genes on and off.

6

Nutrients That Protect DNA from Damage

In recent years, the term "antioxidant," once the province of chemists, has practically become a household word. Most people understand that antioxidant nutrients are good for health because they reduce the risk of disease, primarily by slowing the accumulation of age-related cell damage to the body. Antioxidants accomplish this by preventing free-radical-induced oxidation, the same process that turns iron to rust.

Antioxidants also serve many *non*antioxidant functions. Of particular relevance, they turn some genes on and off, thereby influencing the normal growth of cells as well as protecting against inflammation, cancer, and heart disease. In addition, antioxidants function as cofactors in myriad biochemical reactions and sometimes provide structural roles in cells. The best-known antioxidants are vitamins E and C, but other important ones include carotenoids (such as lutein, lycopene, and beta-carotene), flavonoids (such as quercetin and hesperidin), selenium, N-acetylcysteine, and alpha-lipoic acid.

Most antioxidant research has focused on how these nutrients quench, or neutralize, harmful molecules called free radicals. As discussed in chapter 2, free radicals are unbalanced molecules that lack one electron in what is normally a pair. As a consequence free radicals try to restore their equilibrium by taking a replacement electron from any nearby molecule, such as DNA. By taking that electron, free radicals damage the molecules forming DNA or other cell structures.

Free-radical damage to DNA is disastrous because it can disable or rewrite a cell's genetic programming, which is what happens with cancer cells. Antioxidants neutralize free radicals by donating electrons, which stabilizes them. By protecting against free-radical damage to cells, antioxidants lower the risk of cancer, heart disease, and nearly all diseases.

Free Radicals, Antioxidants, and Your Genes

Both antioxidants and free radicals turn many important genes on and off. Both are necessary, but they generally have opposing effects.

Free Radicals and Stress Genes

Although free radicals can and often do damage genes, they also turn on many genes that initially help protect us from harm. Many of these genes, known as stress genes, are involved in the body's responses to serious biological threats, such as physical injuries or infections. For example, free radicals help turn on genes that promote inflammation, a necessary part of the body's immune response. But when the intake of dietary antioxidants is low, these genes do not turn off when they should. Instead the ongoing activity of stress genes helps sustain a long-term inflammatory response, potentially leading to such chronic diseases as arthritis, heart disease, and cancer.

More specifically, free radicals activate several gene-transcription proteins (including nuclear factor kappa beta, activator protein-1, and heat-shock proteins). These proteins turn on certain genes and begin the process of transcribing information in DNA to RNA, which in turn produces proteins or enzymes. While initially protective, these transcription factors turn on genes that promote inflammation, the growth of cancer cells, and the proliferation of viruses (including HIV) in the body.

During inflammatory responses, particularly when they are chronic, the body's reserves of antioxidants, which should help turn off these genes, can become depleted. Large amounts of supplemental antioxidants often ease disease symptoms, speed recovery, or extend life expectancy. These benefits of antioxidants have been demonstrated many times by physicians and in a wide range of clinical studies. For example, several hospital studies have shown that supplemental antioxidants can quell the immune overreaction that often kills patients with an infection of the blood.

Antioxidants Turn On Helpful Genes in Brain Cells

Only in recent years have scientists begun to discover how antioxidants turn on many important genes. One of the most fascinating studies was conducted by Peter G. Schultz, Ph.D., of the Scripps Research Institute. Schultz and his colleagues gave an extract of the herb ginkgo biloba, which is especially rich in antioxidant compounds, to laboratory mice and then compared the responses of genes in their brain cells to those of mice that had not received ginkgo. This study is significant for two reasons. First, ginkgo is widely used to improve memory, and some research shows that it may slow the progression of Alzheimer's disease. Also, this particular study demonstrated that ginkgo improves the activity of many different genes in brain cells.

Schulz found that ten key genes affecting brain function increased in activity by three to sixteen times after the mice consumed ginkgo. One of the genes increased activity in the hippocampus, the brain's center of learning and memory. The other nine genes positively influenced biochemical activity in the cerebral cortex, which controls memory, speech, logical and emotional responses, and voluntary physical movements. These genetic changes underlie the more obvious improvements in cognition and memory that occur after taking ginkgo.

Antioxidants Disable Genes in Cancer Cells

Antioxidants also help regulate the "cell cycle," which is comparable to a biological clock that regulates cell growth, the replication of DNA, and the creation of new cells. Nearly all cells have a built-in suicide program, called apoptosis. When cells reach a certain age, this suicide program literally stops the clock, triggering the cell's death and preventing its genetic program from turning cancerous. This is a normal process, and the immune system cleans up and disposes of dead cells.

However, cancer cells typically lack this suicide program and do not die until their host dies. In fact, some of the cancer cells used experimentally by researchers are the descendants of cells obtained during surgery on patients decades ago! The genetic programs in cancer cells enable them to be virtually immortal.

Yet researchers have found, time and again in cell and animal studies, that antioxidants can interrupt the life cycle of cancer cells and induce apoptosis. Many of these studies have used natural vitamin E succinate, beta-carotene, and silymarin (an antioxidant extract of the herb milk thistle). In one of these studies, researchers at the AMC Cancer Research Center in Denver found that silymarin stopped the growth of breast-cancer cells just before they were about to replicate DNA for a new cancer cell. None of these nutrients has been found to cause apoptosis in healthy cells, suggesting that they have normal roles in regulating healthy DNA.

Protecting DNA from Free-Radical Damage

Dozens of studies have demonstrated that antioxidants can reduce free-radical damage to DNA, genes, and chromosomes. Let's look briefly at three of them.

In the first study, researchers at the University of Ulster in Northern Ireland exposed cells to various dosages of X-ray radiation or hydrogen peroxide, both generators of free radicals. Some of the cells were also exposed to vitamin C or to vitamin E. Each vitamin protected against DNA damage, but in different ways. Vitamin C did a better job of preventing DNA damage from X-rays, whereas vitamin E was more effective in preventing DNA damage from hydrogen peroxide. Each vitamin quenched free radicals in a different place in the cells.

In the second study, European researchers asked 57 healthy men to take an antioxidant combination or a placebo for twelve weeks. The antioxidant dosages were relatively modest: 149 IU of vitamin E, 100 mg of vitamin C, 6 mg of beta-carotene, and 50 mcg of selenium. The researchers drew blood from the subjects at the beginning and end of the study, and they investigated the amount of genetic damage in the men's lymphocyte cells.

Overall, men taking the antioxidants benefited from more than a 50 percent decrease in genetic damage. Among smokers antioxidants decreased the amount of chromosome damage by almost seven times. A separate group of men, all of whom had survived a heart attack, did not have a decrease in genetic damage from the antioxidants, possibly because their ill health created much higher requirements for these nutrients.

In the third study, researchers looked at genetic damage in workers who had helped clean up the radioactive Chernobyl nuclear power plant. Because of their exposure to radiation, these men had genetic damage ten times higher than normal. But after the men took ginkgo supplements, their genetic damage (measured in the subjects' blood cells) declined to almost normal levels. When the men stopped taking the ginkgo supplements, about one-third of them had an increase in genetic damage, indicating that they needed continued supplementation.

Antioxidant Synergy

The antioxidants that protect us and limit free-radical damage come from two sources, and both are intertwined. Our bodies make a number of antioxidant enzymes, including various glutathione compounds (such as glutathione peroxidase), superoxide dismutase, and catalase. These antioxidants are produced to quench as many free radicals as possible close to their origin, so they do not cause much damage.

Meanwhile, vegetables, fruits, and herbs provide the lion's share of dietary antioxidants. As beneficial as antioxidant supplements are, they should usually be considered just that—supplements to a wholesome diet. Vegetables, fruits, and herbs contain thousands of different antioxidants, most in families of compounds called polyphenols, flavonoids, and carotenoids, which will be discussed later in this chapter.

Unfortunately, companies sometimes advertise that a "super-antioxidant" product is fifty or a hundred times more powerful than vitamins E or C. Such ads are misleading. No single antioxidant can neutralize all types of free radicals. Different antioxidants work in different places in the cell, some are fat-soluble and others water-soluble, and each quenches different types of free radicals. In other words, you and your genes are best served with multiple antioxidants, not just one.

In addition, many antioxidants also interact with each other, supporting each other as they quench free radicals. Lester Packer, Ph.D., professor emeritus of the University of California at Berkeley, has described this antioxidant synergy as the "antioxidant network." For example, alpha-lipoic acid helps restore vitamins C and E and glutathione back to full strength after they have lost electrons fighting free radicals. So again it is better to consume a diversity of antioxidants instead of just one.

Vitamin E

Vitamin E is the body's principal fat-soluble antioxidant, meaning that it works in the fatty regions of cells, such as in cell membranes. It has diverse health benefits, among them a reduction in the risk of heart disease, Alzheimer's disease, and some cancers, as well as an easing of pain in rheumatoid arthritis. These benefits are related to the vitamin's role in protecting DNA and other cell structures from free-radical damage, as well as to its role in turning off unhealthy gene activity.

Unfortunately, vitamin E has often suffered from bad press, dating back almost a century to when researchers considered it nothing more than a fertility vitamin for rodents. The medical use of vitamin E began in the 1940s, when Dr. Evan V. Shute and his colleagues in London, Canada, successfully used it to treat gynecological disorders and coronary artery disease. It was not until the 1960s that vitamin E was officially recognized as an essential nutrient in human health, protecting cell membranes from free-radical oxidation.

As an antioxidant, vitamin E prevents the free-radical oxidation of low-density lipoprotein (LDL) cholesterol, an early step in the development of heart disease. Globules of oxidized LDL (but not normal LDL) trigger an inflammatory response, prompting white blood cells to seek and engulf it. These white blood cells (fattened with oxidized LDL) then stick to artery walls, intensifying a localized inflammatory response. (For more information on this, please see my book *The Inflammation Syndrome.*)

LDL is widely considered the "bad" form of cholesterol. But this is a misconception. LDL carries vitamin E and other fat-soluble antioxidants, such as the carotenoids, through the blood. Normal LDL does not promote cardiovascular disease, and oxidized LDL is actually a reflection of inadequate antioxidant intake. Reducing LDL oxidation, on a long-term basis, is one of the ways vitamin E reduces the risk of heart disease.

During the development of heart disease, a combination of free radicals and oxidized LDL stimulates genes that promote the growth of smooth muscle cells in the arteries. These smooth muscle cells become part of the matrix forming arterial plaque, which also includes cholesterol, white blood cells, and a variety of inflammatory molecules. Vitamin E (as well as vitamin C) inhibits the activity of these genes and prevents the abnormal proliferation of smooth muscle cells.

Vitamin E reduces the risk of heart disease in other ways as well. It is a mild anticoagulant, or blood thinner. Contrary to common medical opinion, it does not increase the anticoagulant effect of warfarin (Coumadin).

Many of the benefits of vitamin E are related to its ability to inhibit gene-transcription factors, such as nuclear factor kappa beta, which turns on inflammation-promoting genes. The natural form of vitamin E reduces blood levels of C-reactive protein, a marker and promoter of inflammation, by 30 to 50 percent. In addition, vitamin E supplements reduce pain and improve mobility in patients with rheumatoid arthritis, another testament to its antiinflammatory properties.

Vitamin E has also been shown to reduce the accumulation of beta-amyloid protein in the brain, one of the hallmarks of Alzheimer's disease. Free radicals stimulate the formation of beta-amyloid protein, and it is very likely that this activity involves regulation of the genes that code for beta-amyloid protein, not just a simple free-radical and antioxidant interaction. Several human studies have found that people who consume large amounts of vitamin E have a relatively low risk of developing Alzheimer's disease, and one study found that large amounts of vitamin E slowed the progression of Alzheimer's disease.

How to Take Vitamin E Supplements

For the most part, natural and synthetic vitamins are indistinguishable from each other, but this is not the case with vitamin E. The natural and synthetic forms of vitamin E have different molecular and chemical characteristics. The natural form is more potent and is absorbed twice as well as the synthetic form.

You can easily identify the natural and synthetic forms in supplements, but you have to read the fine print on the back of the label. Natural vitamin E will be identified by its chemical name, d-alpha tocopherol, d-alpha tocopheryl acetate, or d-alpha tocopheryl succinate. Synthetic forms will have a "dl" instead of a "d" before the rest of the chemical name. Companies that do not list either "dl" or "d" on labels are most likely trying to hide the source of their product, which is probably synthetic.

Some natural vitamin E products also contain other forms of vitamin E, such as gamma tocopherol and a vitamin E subfamily of compounds called tocotrienols. Virtually all of the research on vitamin E has been on the d-alpha form, and the body preferentially selects this form for absorption. However, the other forms of vitamin E have antioxidant properties and are also beneficial in conjunction with the d-alpha forms of vitamin E. I take a natural "mixed tocopherol" supplement to get the benefits of full-spectrum vitamin E. Perhaps the best selection of natural vitamin E products is sold by Carlson Laboratories, (800) 323-4141.

How much should you take? Follow these guidelines:

* To reduce DNA damage and your long-term risk of heart disease, cancer, and Alzheimer's disease, take 200 to 400 IU of vitamin E daily. This is a beneficial dose when taken in conjunction with other antioxidants discussed in this chapter.
* To complement the treatment of heart disease, Alzheimer's disease, cancer, and rheumatoid arthritis, take 1,000 to 2,000 IU of vitamin E daily. However, work with your physician in these instances.

Mysterious Symptoms Caused by Celiac Disease

Claire, age forty-five, had suffered from iron-deficiency anemia most of her life, despite taking a daily multivitamin supplement and extra iron. After she had experienced fractures on three different occasions, a bone scan found that she was suffering from osteoporosis, which was unusual for a perimenopausal woman. Over the next year, Claire took still more iron supplements and also calcium supplements, but follow-up tests indicated that she was still anemic and her bones even thinner.

A nutritionally oriented physician suspected that Claire had celiac disease, an intolerance of gluten protein in wheat, barley, and rye. He ordered two tests: a genetic test for the presence of the HLA-DQ2 gene, which is often seen in people with celiac disease, and antitissue transglutaminase, a frequent marker of gluten sensitivity. The doctor's hunch was correct. Both tests came back positive.

The most common form of celiac disease involves an immune response that often quietly attacks the intestinal wall, reducing absorption of many different nutrients. Both iron-deficiency anemia and osteoporosis are observed in people with celiac disease. But often the health consequences of celiac disease go unnoticed for years.

Claire's physician put her in touch with a nutritionist and a celiac support group. The only treatment is the complete avoidance of all gluten-containing food products, which includes most breads, pastas, and processed foods. Although many celiac patients enjoy high-carb gluten-free breads and snacks, Claire has found that a nutrient-dense diet (as described in chapter 7) was the best way for her to avoid gluten.

Her diet includes chicken, turkey, fish, pork, and vegetables— but no bread or other grains, except for a little brown rice. In addition, she takes a high-potency vitamin and a mineral supplement to make up for years of marginal nutrient absorption. To her pleasant surprise, Claire has lost fifteen pounds and a skin condition has also cleared up.

Vitamin C

Our biological ancestors made their own vitamin C, and today most mammals, including dogs and cats, still do. But humans, higher primates (including gorillas and orangutans), and a small number of other animals cannot. We still have the genes that program the synthesis of vitamin C from glucose, but the gene that codes for the final enzyme in the process is damaged in all humans and thus nonfunctional, most likely because of an ancient virus.

Vitamin C–producing animals make the human equivalent of about 1 to 13 grams of vitamin C daily, and these levels increase when the animal is under stress. In contrast, vitamin C levels in humans are quickly depleted by stress. (A physician friend related that after the stress of a spider bite, blood tests showed that his levels of vitamin C were undetectable for days.) If you think of vitamin C as an abundant and endogenously produced substance, like the thousands of other biochemicals made in the body, it becomes clear that even the best diets leave us with only marginal vitamin C levels.

In addition to its antioxidant function, vitamin C appears to be part of the body's stress response and helps us maintain homeostasis, a state of biochemical and metabolic balance. The vitamin is needed for the synthesis of adrenaline (one of our stress hormones), and it also enhances our mood and general sense of well-being. The first signs of vitamin C deficiency are irritability and fatigue.

Considerable research has shown that vitamin C, like vitamin E, reduces free-radical damage to DNA. However, vitamin C appears to play a far more fundamental role in regulating genes and cell growth. Dr. Richard T. Lee of the Harvard Medical School tested 880 chemical compounds to see if any of them prompted embryonic stem cells— essentially generic cells—to differentiate into more specialized heart cells. Such differentiation and specialization of cells enable a few embryonic stem cells to develop into a fetus. In Lee's experiments only vitamin C triggered this transformation from generic cells to heart cells. He wrote with amazement in the journal *Circulation* that the heart cells even pulsated! Thus, vitamin C plays a crucial role in creating new and replacing old cells in the body, and it can do this only by regulating the activity of DNA in embryonic stem cells.

In 1970, the Nobel laureate Linus Pauling, Ph.D., stirred considerable controversy by recommending large amounts of vitamin C to prevent and treat the common cold and influenza. Since then many studies have shown that regular supplemental vitamin C intake, in the range of 2 to 6 grams (2,000 to 6,000 mg) daily, does in fact reduce cold symptoms. In a review article, Harri Hemilä, Ph.D., a professor at the University of Helsinki, analyzed twenty-one vitamin C studies and found that supplemental vitamin C reduced cold symptoms and duration by about one-third.

Although Hemilä published his analysis in 1994, more recent studies have confirmed his findings. If you are fighting an infection, your vitamin C requirements (for immune cells, healing, and homeostasis) increase considerably. Dr. Robert Cathcart III, of Los Altos, California, has long recommended "bowel tolerance" to gauge vitamin C needs, which will change during the course of a cold or flu. Cathcart has suggested that people take enough vitamin C (in divided daily dosages) to the point where they almost develop diarrhea, then reduce the amount to what creates soft stools. That, he believes, is a person's ideal dosage.

Several studies have found that modest dosages (500 mg) of vitamin C can lead to substantial reductions in blood pressure among people with mild to moderate hypertension. Some research also suggests that vitamin C can reduce the risk of stroke, most likely because it is involved in maintaining the integrity of blood vessels. Vitamin C functions as a cofactor in the body's production of collagen and other proteins in tissues, and low levels of the vitamin prevent DNA from fulfilling its normal function in making these proteins.

Pauling raised another controversy when he recommended that cancer patients take a minimum of 10 grams of vitamin C daily. His initial work in this area yielded inconsistent results. However, Canada's Dr. Abram Hoffer has developed a high-potency anticancer vitamin program around Pauling's initial recommendations, and he has had great success in treating cancer and preventing the recurrence of cancer in hundreds of patients. Dr. Mark Levine of the National Institutes of

Health has noted that intravenous vitamin C may be more effective than oral supplements in treating cancer. The reason is that intravenous vitamin C is more effective than oral supplements at raising blood levels.

Several studies have found that people with high intake or high blood levels of vitamin C live longer than people who consume little of the vitamin. In one recent study, Dr. Kay-Tee Khaw of Cambridge University found that people with high blood levels of vitamin C had half the risk of death at any age, compared with those who had low levels of vitamin C.

Finally, several studies have shown that the topical application of lotions with vitamin C can reduce the depth of wrinkles and improve overall skin tone. This research is significant because it demonstrates that some signs of aging, aged cells, and DNA and cell-membrane damage can be partially reversed.

How to Take Vitamin C Supplements

It is easy to feel overwhelmed by the many different types of vitamin C supplements on the market. Ascorbic acid is the chemical name for vitamin C, and this type is generally the least expensive. However, pay careful attention to the excipients listed in the fine print. Excipients are substances, including cellulose, lactose, sugar, and colorings that are added to improve the manufacturing, taste, or appearance of tablets and capsules. In general, supplements (of all types) sold in health and natural food stores have fewer excipients and smaller quantities than supplements sold in drugstores.

- Most people should take a minimum of 500 to 1,000 mg of vitamin C daily. Whatever the dosage you take, it is best to divide it up and take smaller amounts two or three times daily.
- An ideal dosage range is 2,000 to 5,000 mg a day, again divided up two or three times daily.
- You may need higher dosages, particularly if you are fighting a cold or flu.
- If you develop loose stools or diarrhea, you are taking too much vitamin C. Use the "bowel tolerance" method to adjust your vitamin C dosage. Reduce the amount to slightly less than what it takes to cause loose stools. This amount is your ideal dosage.
- It is also worthwhile to add some type of flavonoid supplement (see "Flavonoids" later in this chapter). Flavonoids work with vitamin C, and the two have synergistic benefits.

Selenium

Selenium, an essential dietary mineral, is a component of the body's four glutathione peroxidase compounds, among the most powerful antioxidants made by the body.

In a recent study, German and Italian researchers found that a particular selenium-containing enzyme, phospholipid hydroperoxide glutathione peroxidase, is produced in large quantities in developing sperm, where it protects against free-radical damage to DNA. However, the function of this enzyme changes as sperm mature, and it provides some of the physical structure of sperm.

In a series of animal experiments and human studies, Melinda Beck, Ph.D., of the University of North Carolina at Chapel Hill found that selenium can curb the spread of flu and coxsackie viruses. In contrast, selenium deficiency actually spurs their activity.

These viruses, along with the AIDS and Ebola viruses, use selenium-containing proteins to reproduce. During an infection the viruses deplete the body's reserves of selenium, which impairs the production of glutathione peroxidase and the body's immune response to the infection. Intuitively, you might think that depriving the viruses of selenium would help stop them. But that is not the case. Several studies have found that selenium deficiency leads to specific mutations in the flu and coxsackie viruses, which make the viruses far more dangerous. Once the viral mutation is created, it can even infect a healthy person who consumes adequate selenium.

The solution is to maintain adequate intake of selenium, which boosts the immune system's ability to fight the virus and to either destroy it or keep it in check. Small studies on patients with AIDS have found that supplemental selenium can control viral replication and extend life expectancy.

Selenium supplements can also reduce the risk of several types of cancer. Through its role in glutathione peroxidases, selenium likely helps prevent DNA mutations that would give rise to cancer cells. The late Larry C. Clark, Ph.D., of the University of Arizona found that people who took 200 mcg of selenium daily had a 63 percent lower risk of prostate cancer, a 58 percent lower risk of colorectal cancer, and a 46 percent lower risk of lung cancer. These are impressive results from taking a single supplement daily for only a few years.

Recently, Dr. Rebecca E. Rudolph of the Fred Hutchinson Cancer Research Center in Seattle linked high selenium levels to a lower risk of Barrett's esophagus. The condition, a complication of chronic heart-burn, boosts the risk of esophageal cancer by seventy-five times. Rudolph found that patients with high blood levels of selenium had about half the risk of developing precancerous cell changes in the esophagus. Selenium helps maintain normal functioning of the p53 cancer-suppressing gene, which is damaged or not active in many cancers.

How to Take Selenium Supplements

There are many high-quality selenium supplements on the market. My personal preference is for a high-selenium yeast supplement (in which yeast is grown in a selenium-rich environment and then harvested). However, you cannot go wrong with other types of selenium supplements.

- Taking 200 mcg daily (which may already be in your multivitamin supplement) is safe and can reduce the risk of several different types of cancer.
- If you have frequent colds and flus or chronic infections (such as HIV or hepatitis C), take 400 mcg daily.

Carotenoids

Carotenoids are a family of fat-soluble pigments that add color to vegetables and fruits. As antioxidants they protect plants from free radicals, which are generated when ultraviolet rays (in sunlight) strike the plants. When we consume plants as part of our diet, we acquire many of the antioxidant benefits of carotenoids.

In addition, carotenoids influence the expression of some genes in plants and appear to influence the behavior of some genes in people. Carotenoids also play key roles in what scientists call "gap junction communication." Gap junctions span the physical gaps between cells and, as the term suggests, they enable one cell to communicate with its neighboring cells. It is through such communication that cells share information about conditions and also whether certain genes should be activated.

More than six hundred carotenoids have been identified, but only about twenty are absorbed from foods in the diet. Of these, beta-carotene, lutein, and lycopene are the most common and probably most important in terms of health.

Beta-Carotene

Beta-carotene, perhaps the best known of all carotenoids, functions as an antioxidant that protects against free-radical damage to DNA. Considerable research supports this benefit of beta-carotene. In one study, published in the *European Journal of Nutrition*, researchers found that people taking 15 mg of natural beta-carotene daily reduced DNA damage and enhanced DNA repair.

Beta-carotene also influences the activity of a key cancer-suppressing gene, known as p21. This gene programs the structure of the p21 protein. Lucia A. Stivala, Ph.D., and her colleagues at the University of Pavia in Italy conducted research showing that some of the anticancer properties of beta-carotene are related to its effect on the p21 gene. In experiments Stivala found that beta-carotene inhibited the growth of skin-cancer cells but only in the presence of the p21 gene. Other research has shown that vitamin E increases the activity of the p21 gene, leading to large amounts of the p21 protein, suggesting that vitamin E and beta-carotene influence gene behavior in tandem, apart from their joint antioxidant activity.

In the colon, dietary fiber indirectly also increases the activity of the p21 gene. Fiber is not absorbed, but it is fermented by bacteria while passing through the intestine. This fermentation produces butyrate, a compound that turns on the p21 gene. Experiments have found that active p21 genes actually turn off a separate gene that promotes the growth of colon-cancer cells.

Some research has shown that people who smoke more than a pack of cigarettes daily and also drink substantial amounts of alcohol (spirits) have a slightly higher risk of developing lung cancer if they also take synthetic beta-carotene supplements. Smoking and alcohol generate large numbers of free radicals and cause genetic damage throughout the body. The combination overwhelms the antioxidant benefits of beta-carotene and, ironically, creates more free radicals from beta-carotene. Because of these findings, heavy smokers and drinkers should not take synthetic beta-carotene.

However, studies have clearly shown that former smokers and nondrinkers do benefit from beta-carotene and have a lower risk of developing lung cancer when taking supplements. In addition, several studies suggest that a combination of antioxidants, including natural beta-carotene, is associated with a lower risk of lung cancer. Natural beta-carotene supplements are preferable to the synthetic form, because they contain some alpha-carotene, which appears to protect against lung cancer. So the best advice should be the most obvious: don't smoke tobacco or drink excessive amounts of alcohol, because no supplement will totally erase their negative health consequences.

Health problems have never been associated with the carotenoids in foods. Carrots, pumpkins, and other vegetables are excellent sources of beta-carotene and other carotenoids.

Lycopene

Lycopene, a red carotenoid found in tomatoes and watermelon, concentrates in the prostate and can reduce the risk of prostate cancer. In one study, researchers from the Harvard School of Public Health reported that high intake of tomato sauces, rich in lycopene and related carotenoids, reduced the risk of prostate cancer by 45 percent. Still other research has found strong associations between high intake of lycopene (or tomatoes) and a low risk of other cancers, including those of the pancreas, colon, breast, and cervix.

Like beta-carotene, lycopene appears to function both as an antioxidant and as a regulator of some genes. For example, lycopene inhibits the activity of "transforming growth factor alpha," which alters gene behavior and stimulates the growth of cancers.

Some human evidence suggests that lycopene interrupts the growth of prostate-cancer cells, and this would likely take place through apoptosis, which involves shutting down DNA replication. A team of doctors from the Karmano Cancer Institute in Detroit gave 30 mg of lycopene or a placebo daily to 36 men scheduled for prostate-cancer surgery. After three weeks tumors in the men taking lycopene had shrunk significantly and their cancer cells showed a reduced tendency toward proliferation. This does not mean that lycopene is a cure for prostate cancer. However, one cannot help but wonder whether the men might have benefited from further cancer remission if they had taken the supplements for several months.

Lutein and Zeaxanthin

Lutein and zeaxanthin, found in kale, spinach, and broccoli, also serve as antioxidant carotenoids. They are deposited in the macula, the center of the eye's retina, responsible for detailed vision. These yellowish deposits of lutein and zeaxanthin are referred to as the macular pigment, and they help filter out harmful wavelengths of light. This area of pigment, smaller than the head of a pin, also functions somewhat like a pair of polarized sunglasses, improving visual acuity in bright situations.

A thin layer of macular pigment is a prime risk factor for macular degeneration, the leading (and generally untreatable) cause of blindness in the elderly. Supplemental lutein, some of which the body converts to zeaxanthin, increases the thickness of the macular pigment and can often improve visual acuity in people with macular degeneration and retinitis pigmentosa, an inherited eye disease.

How to Take Carotenoid Supplements

The best source of carotenoids is a diet rich in fruits and colorful, non-starchy vegetables. If you opt for supplements, it is important to obtain a combination of beta-carotene, lycopene, and lutein. Natural beta-carotene (from algae) is superior to the synthetic form. Natural tomato-derived lycopene contains related carotenoids that are likely of value, but synthetic lycopene may be an alternative for people with tomato or nightshade-plant sensitivities. Lutein is extracted from marigold petals and is sold as pure (or "free") lutein and as lutein esters. Both products are natural, well absorbed, and functionally equivalent.

- For most people supplemental daily dosages should be approximately 6 mg (10,000 IU) of beta-carotene, 5 mg of lycopene, and 5 mg of lutein.
- Higher dosages may offset specific health risks, such as benign prostate enlargement or cancer (30 mg of lycopene) or macular degeneration (20 mg of lutein).

An Improved Diet and Supplements Reverse Jared's Prediabetes

Like many men, Jared enjoyed eating pizza and drinking beer, and he had a sweet tooth as well. By the time he turned forty-five, he had a sizable potbelly. He was thirty pounds overweight and had a forty-inch waist. A blood test showed that his fasting glucose was 105 mg/dl, his fasting insulin was 38 mcIU/ml, and his glycated hemoglobin was 8.5 percent, together indicating that he would probably be diagnosed with type 2 diabetes within the next few years.

The prospect of diabetes was a wake-up call for Jared. His physician explained that elevated glucose and insulin levels turn on genes that promote obesity, heart disease, kidney disease, and possibly even some types of cancer. Because Jared's father had died of diabetic complications, he was especially motivated to avoid a similar fate.

In conjunction with his nutritionally oriented physician and a nutritionist, Jared worked hard to modify his diet, eating more chicken, fish, steamed vegetables, and salads. He stopped drinking beer and instead started drinking mineral water and tea. He began taking antioxidant supplements, including vitamins E and C and alpha-lipoic acid, all of which have been shown to improve glucose tolerance. In addition, he also began going for long walks—two to three miles daily—which his physician said would also help lower his glucose and insulin levels.

Six months later Jared had lost 30 pounds and achieved his target weight of 150 pounds. He felt better than he had in years and understood that he was not just on a diet but was improving his dietary habits for the rest of his life. A year later blood tests showed that his fasting glucose had dropped to 86, his insulin to 10, and his glycated hemoglobin to 6.1 percent. Excited by his makeover, Jared plans to further improve his health and bring these numbers down even more.

Flavonoids

Like carotenoids, flavonoids (sometimes called polyphenolic flavonoids and bioflavonoids) function as pigments and antioxidants in plants. They also influence some gene activity in plants, suggesting that they may do the same in people. We obtain the antioxidant benefits of flavonoids when we eat vegetables and fruits, and tantalizing research suggests that they have positive effects on our genes as well. Studies have found that people who consume large amounts of flavonoids have a relatively low risk of cancer. Flavonoids turn on protective genes, turn off inflammation-promoting genes, and protect against gene-damaging free radicals.

To the surprise of many people, flavonoids account for most of the antioxidants in vegetables and fruits. More than five thousand individual flavonoids have been identified in plants, and scientists have organized flavonoids into several large families based on their chemical structure. From the standpoint of health benefits, a few specific flavonoids are of interest.

Anthocyanidins

Anthocyanidins are a family of dark-colored flavonoids concentrated in blueberries, raspberries, certain herbs, purple grapes, and red wines. Two flavonoid supplements, Pycnogenol and grapeseed extract, are rich in anthocyanidins. Pycnogenol is obtained from the bark of French maritime pine trees, whereas grapeseed extract is derived from waste material in the wine industry. Both supplements contain complexes of many individual antioxidant flavonoids, with some similarities and differences.

Experiments have shown that Pycnogenol reduces the activity of two genes, calgranulin A and B, by twenty-two times in skin cells. These two genes are overactive in psoriasis and other skin diseases, and so Pycnogenol may be beneficial in psoriasis. Other research has found that Pycnogenol protects against some of the harmful effects of ultraviolet (UV) rays in sunlight. In these experiments researchers used UV rays to turn on genes involved in inflammation following sunburn. Cells exposed to Pycnogenol maintained lower gene activity after being exposed to UV rays.

Pycnogenol also appears to regulate the gene that codes for nitric oxide synthase, an enzyme involved in the production of nitric oxide. Nitric oxide is a key gene-regulating molecule. Viagra and the other prescription drugs for erectile dysfunction work by increasing nitric oxide levels. One study found Pycnogenol helpful in erectile dysfunction as well.

Citrus Flavonoids

Lemons, limes, oranges, grapefruit, and other citrus fruits are rich sources of flavonoids. Most of these flavonoids are found in the internal membranes of the fruits and in the bitter rind.

Cell studies have found that a flavonoid called naringin, found principally in grapefruit, can protect bone-cell chromosomes from radiation damage. This characteristic, if true in humans, would lower the risk of leukemia. Other studies have found that naringenin, a closely related compound, can inhibit the growth of colon- and breast-cancer cells.

In a human study, German researchers used large dosages of the flavonoid limonene, found in lemons and oranges, to treat women with breast cancer. Tumor growth was inhibited in some but not all of the patients, a promising finding. The researchers gave 13.8 grams of limonene daily to the women in the study. Fresh lemonade, made from whole lemons, provides 1 gram of limonene per liter, but commercial juices provide only about one-twelfth that amount.

Cell studies have shown that many other citrus flavonoids likely protect against cancer. Among them are hesperidin, luteolin, and diosmin, all found in lemons and oranges. They appear to work by interfering with the life cycle of cancer cells, thereby destroying them. Flavonoids do not have this destructive effect on normal cells.

Flavonoids in Herbs and Spices

Most of the antioxidants and other biologically active compounds found in ginkgo biloba and other herbs are flavonoids or members of their parent chemical family, polyphenols. In fact, approximately a thousand chemical compounds have been identified in ginkgo, a sharp contrast to single-molecule pharmaceutical drugs.

Many of the compounds found in ginkgo, St. John's wort, ginseng, and other herbs are also found in vegetables and fruits. However, other compounds are highly distinctive and found only in certain herbs, such as the ginkolides in ginkgo and the ginsenosides in ginseng.

How to Take Flavonoid Supplements

As with carotenoids, the best way to obtain a diverse selection of flavonoids is by eating a diet with a healthy range of vegetables and fruits. The reason is simple: no supplement can provide the variety of flavonoids found in foods.

- People at risk of inflammatory diseases, heart disease, or cancer may wish to take extra flavonoids in the form of supplements. Consider taking 50 to 200 mg of either Pycnogenol or grapeseed extract, or 500 to 1,000 mg of citrus flavonoids, daily.
- To reduce inflammation, strive for 200 mg of either Pycnogenol or grapeseed extract. Consider trying both to see which works best for you.

N-Acetylcysteine

N-acetylcysteine (NAC) is part of a family of sulfur-containing antioxidants known to chemists as thiols. In one of the paradoxes of nutritional science, sulfur has been virtually ignored as an essential nutrient. Yet we would not be able to live without it. Sulfur compounds help hold our tissues together and are also part of several amino acids (such as methionine, cysteine, and taurine, which DNA requires to execute its functions) insulin, and some B vitamins.

NAC is rich in both sulfur and the amino acid cysteine. As a supplement it is preferable to pure cysteine, which may be neurotoxic in high dosages. In contrast, large amounts of NAC are safe. NAC serves as a precursor to various glutathione compounds, the most powerful antioxidants made within the body.

NAC is considered a "chemopreventive" compound because it can lower the risk of cancer. The cancer-protective effects of NAC have been documented for more than thirty-five years. Some of NAC's anticancer benefits can be attributed to its ability to increase protective glutathione levels. But many properties of NAC are distinctive. For example, NAC can block some of the chemical signals that tell cancer cells to grow.

NAC is also a powerful immune stimulant, protecting against viral infections. Lenora Herzenberg, Ph.D., Leonard Herzenberg, Ph.D., and their colleagues at Stanford University reported that large dosages of NAC—3,200 to 8,000 mg daily—for six weeks significantly boosted glutathione levels in subjects with AIDS. People who continued taking NAC had a significantly increased rate of survival.

NAC also protects against flu symptoms, probably more effectively than does vitamin C. Dr. Silvio De Flora of the University of Genoa asked 262 elderly subjects to take either 600 mg of NAC or a placebo daily for six months over the wintertime cold and flu season. Although NAC did not prevent them from contracting the flu, it had a striking effect on symptoms. Of the subjects who had a laboratory-confirmed flu, only 25 percent of those taking NAC developed symptoms. In contrast, 79 percent of those taking the placebo had obvious and uncomfortable flu symptoms, according to De Flora's article in the *European Respiratory Journal*. In other words, NAC supplements reduced the likelihood of having flu symptoms by more than two-thirds.

Of particular interest is the fact that garlic contains many sulfur-based antioxidants very similar to NAC. This similarity to NAC may account for garlic's many reputed benefits.

How to Take NAC Supplements

NAC is exceptionally safe as a dietary supplement. NAC capsules, however, possess a rotten-egg smell because of the sulfur content. So it is wise to resist the temptation to smell NAC supplements and, instead, simply to swallow them.

- For general health maintenance, take 500 mg of NAC daily. Double this amount during the cold and flu season.
- When fighting infections you may need to take 2,000 to 3,000 mg of NAC daily. These higher dosages work best when started on the first day of the cold or flu.

Alpha-Lipoic Acid

Alpha-lipoic acid, which plays key roles in the production of cellular energy (see chapter 4), is also a potent and versatile antioxidant. Like NAC, it contains sulfur and is a precursor to glutathione compounds. As an antioxidant, it protects against nerve damage in diabetes, and it also improves the transmission of nerve signals in diabetic neuropathy and sciatica. As discussed earlier, it reduces the activity of transcription proteins that turn on genes involved in inflammation, replication of the human immunodeficiency virus, and cancer growth.

Alpha-lipoic acid has some distinctive antioxidant properties. For one thing, the body converts some alpha-lipoic acid to dihydrolipoic acid, which is an even more powerful antioxidant. Alpha-lipoic acid also functions in both fat-containing and water-containing cell regions. This quality is in contrast to most other antioxidants, which work in one place or the other but not both.

Together, alpha-lipoic acid and dihydrolipoic acid neutralize a wide variety of DNA-damaging free radicals. For example, alpha-lipoic acid quenches hydroxyl free radicals—the most dangerous type—whereas dihydrolipoic acid protects against peroxyl and peroxynitrite free radicals.

Alpha-lipoic acid possesses still one more distinctive quality as an antioxidant: it helps recycle several other antioxidants. Typically, antioxidants become weak (harmless) free radicals after quenching destructive free radicals. Alpha-lipoic acid donates electrons to other antioxidants, helping return vitamins C and E, glutathione, and coenzyme Q10 back to full strength. By restoring their antioxidant capacity, alpha-lipoic acid extends the ability of these antioxidants to fight free radicals.

How to Take Alpha-Lipoic Acid Supplements

For simple antioxidant protection, 50 to 100 mg of alpha-lipoic acid should be sufficient. European sources of alpha-lipoic acid tend to be of higher quality than those from Asia, so it is wise to inquire about where a company purchases the raw material for its alpha-lipoic acid supplements. For specific conditions, refer to the discussion of alpha-lipoic acid in chapter 4.

In the following section, we will focus on eating plans that foster normal gene function and reduce the risk of disease.

PART III

Gene-Enhancing Eating Plans

7

Dietary Guidelines for Feeding Your Genes Right

When people talk about "going on" a particular diet, their choice of words implies that they will in time go off it. In other words, they temporarily change what they eat, achieve their objectives, and then return to their previous and unhealthy eating patterns. This situation explains why many people on weight-reduction diets ultimately regain the weight they lose—they eventually go back to eating the foods that originally made them fat.

A more sensible and long-term approach to healthy eating consists of two steps. The first is modifying your eating habits to reverse or lower the odds of developing health problems, in this case to foster healthy DNA and optimal gene function. The second is maintaining these new eating habits relatively consistently for the rest of your life.

In the course of making dietary changes, it is important that you take one step at a time, while seeing your actions as stepping-stones toward the goal of permanently improving your eating habits. At first it may be hard to imagine making major dietary changes and then adhering to them for the rest of your life. That is why it is so important to adopt the guidelines one or two at a time (although you're certainly free to adopt them faster). If you are reluctant to make changes, I recommend that you follow some of the guidelines in this chapter for just one week, which should be easy. Many people tell me they feel better, have more energy, and are less fuzzy-headed within several days of making these changes. Feeling better is a powerful motivator for continuing, and as time goes on, this way of eating will become second nature to you, just as it has for me.

By following these dietary guidelines, you will create a sound foundation for feeding your genes right, maintaining a healthy weight, improving how you feel on a day-to-day basis, and lowering your long-term risk of disease.

Getting Ready to Change Your Eating Habits

As you read this chapter, you may be thinking, "Easier said than done," and feeling how uncomfortable it is to make changes. Granted, it does take a conscious effort to change your eating habits, but it is actually easier than you might think.

We all know that it is difficult for people to change their habits, particularly eating habits. Our experience has taught us that such changes usually entail giving up some favorite foods or the large portion sizes we enjoy eating. We also are accustomed to certain tastes and smells, to our own personal comfort foods, and we are often wary of different foods, even if they might be healthier.

Getting used to selecting healthier foods in supermarkets and restaurants has a lot in common with starting a new job. There is a learning curve, which may be easy or difficult for you. At the beginning it helps to remember that whatever type of work you do, you did not start out knowing what you now do about your job. On your first day, you most likely began with a hazy idea of what you were supposed to accomplish, and you may have felt uncertain about your abilities and been afraid of failing. These are all normal feelings. But in time you learned how to master your job, and doing it became second nature to you.

The same learning curve and initial emotional uncertainty exist when you initially work to improve your eating habits. At first this job might seem like a daunting task, just as your regular job once did. After all, there is a lot to learn and there are probably a few bad habits to break. But for everything you might have to give up or modify, you will likely discover new and satisfying flavors, as well as a pleasant sense of well-being.

As you continue to improve your diet, some of your attitudes toward food may change also. I'll give you a personal example. I used to be what I now jokingly call a "pastaholic." I enjoyed pasta almost every day, and usually extra helpings. But from a nutritional standpoint, pasta is almost entirely starch—empty calories. After years of regularly eating pasta, I developed an unflattering pot gut, and my fasting blood sugar was creeping toward prediabetic levels.

In early 1999 circumstances in my life interrupted my regular pasta habit for a few days. After a week I tried my favorite pasta dish and found that it did not seem as tasty as it had in the past. As a result I started eating more salads and baked chicken. Over the next three months, I lost twenty pounds and four inches from my waist without consciously trying to lose weight. In addition, my blood-sugar levels dropped twenty-seven points, to within the normal range. I liked how I was looking, and I beamed at how the changes were reflected in my medical tests. In fact, I was able to qualify for a deep discount on a life insurance policy because of how impressively those blood tests demonstrated my better health. Five years later, as I write this book, I have no difficulty maintaining my lower weight, and my overall health seems to be better than ever.

But my changes were not just dietary or physical. My attitude toward food had also changed. I no longer saw pasta as an appetizing dish. Rather, when a plate of pasta went by in a restaurant, it looked like an unappetizing mound of high-calorie carbohydrates. Today I see pasta as an absolute waste of calories that I could better spend on far more interesting and tastier foods. Similarly, I used to enjoy french fries, but I now find the smell of fast food as appealing as a cloud of diesel exhaust from a truck. And when I see people eating candy bars and soft drinks instead of a real lunch, I see them increasing their chances of becoming fat and diabetic.

This preamble to setting forth my dietary guidelines is a way of saying that your attitudes toward food and dietary habits, like mine, can change profoundly—and that you can become very comfortable with these changes. The payoff comes with feeling and looking better and at some point, perhaps a few years in the future, seeing that you do not suffer the health problems afflicting your friends, relatives, and coworkers.

The following twelve nutrition guidelines foster eating habits that provide a nutrient-rich environment for maintaining healthy DNA and normal gene activity. Again, if these guidelines still seem a bit imposing, follow some of them for just one week and then consider how you feel.

—⚋—

Twelve Guidelines for Feeding Your Genes Right

Guideline 1: Eat a nutrient-dense diet to make every bite count.

Guideline 2: Eat a variety of fresh, whole foods.

Guideline 3: Eat quality protein.

Guideline 4: Eat a varied selection of nonstarchy vegetables.

Guideline 5: Eat a varied selection of nonstarchy fruits.

Guideline 6: Consume only healthy oils and fats.

Guideline 7: Season your foods with herbs and spices.

Guideline 8: Drink water and teas.

Guideline 9: Eat organically produced foods whenever possible.

Guideline 10: Restrict or avoid refined carbohydrates and sugars, and limit your intake of all processed carbohydrates.

Guideline 11: Minimize your consumption of highly refined cooking oils.

Guideline 12: Avoid all foods with partially hydrogenated vegetable oils and trans fats.

—⚋—

Guideline 1: Eat a Nutrient-Dense Diet to Make Every Bite Count

Eating a nutrient-dense diet is the single most important dietary guideline for feeding your genes right. This recommendation is the umbrella guideline for most of the others that follow.

What exactly does eating for nutrient density mean? Quite simply, it is striving to obtain the best nutrition—the most vitamins, vitaminlike nutrients, minerals, protein, fiber, and healthy fats—in each calorie you eat. With two-thirds of Americans overweight or obese, and with obesity increasing worldwide, it is of utmost importance to obtain high-quality nutrition in the fewest possible calories. When you eat a nutrient-dense diet, you do not waste calories on "genetically unfamiliar" nutrient-poor foods such as sugars, refined carbohydrates, and unhealthy fats.

For example, a chicken Caesar salad (without croutons) is a nutrient-dense lunch relative to its total calorie content. The chicken provides protein and some vitamins, the greens provide a broad selection of antioxidants and fiber, and the dressing should provide some healthy fats. In contrast, a double-scoop ice cream cone might provide the same number of calories, but its high concentration of sugars, starches, and unhealthy fats does not make it a nutritionally desirable food.

As a general rule, nutrient-dense foods are relatively low in carbohydrates. These foods include fish, chicken, turkey, lean meats, salad greens, tomatoes, broccoli, cauliflower, raspberries, and blueberries. (The fish and chicken should not be breaded or fried.) A nutrient-dense dinner could consist of poached salmon and steamed broccoli because this combination is high in protein, vitamins, minerals, fiber, and healthy fats. If you are physically active or if you do not need to lose weight, you may add a small amount of brown rice or sweet potato to the meal. This particular meal would contain only a small amount of carbohydrate, which is adequate for most people. (See "Some Acceptable High-Carb Foods in Moderation" later in this chapter.)

Why is a nutrient-dense diet healthier for you and your genes? As you learned in chapter 3, the original human diet consisted of nutrient-dense foods, such as animal protein and vegetables. Over many years this nutrient-dense milieu became the de facto environment for our DNA and genes. DNA synthesis and repair and normal gene function became dependent on a rich supply of nutrients but relatively small amounts of carbohydrates.

In contrast, nutrient-poor foods fail to provide adequate amounts of protein, vitamins, vitamin-like nutrients, minerals, fiber, or healthy fats. Their high levels of sugars, carbohydrates, and unhealthy fats stimulate hormonal changes and gene activity that promote inflammation, obesity, diabetes, heart disease, and cancer.

—∞—

How Are These Dietary Guidelines Different from Those of the Atkins Diet or Other High-Protein Diets?

You might be wondering how the dietary recommendations in *Feed Your Genes Right* differ from those of the Atkins diet. The Atkins diet is the most popular high-protein diet, but it has often been criticized for its high levels of saturated fat.

Both the Atkins and the *Feed Your Genes Right* recommendations encourage people to eat more nutrient-dense protein. However, the guidelines in this book emphasize protein sources, such as fish, chicken, and turkey, that are relatively low in saturated fat.

While small to moderate amounts of saturated fat (such as the occasional use of butter or cream) should not pose a problem for most people, large quantities of saturated fats can displace healthier fats from the diet. For example, eating mostly beef or pork leaves limited room for fish, such as salmon, that are high in healthy omega-3 family fats.

Finally, *Feed Your Genes Right* recommends a more balanced overall eating plan that includes large amounts of nutrient-dense, non-starchy vegetables and fruits. The principal restriction is in the quantity of empty carbohydrate calories, such as in breads, pastas, and most other baked items.

—⟋⟍—

Guideline 2: Eat a Variety of Fresh, Whole Foods

Most fresh, whole foods are rich sources of nutrients. In contrast, refined and processed foods usually have their most nutritious components separated and removed as part of large-scale manufacturing processes.

How do you recognize fresh, whole foods? It's simple. Whole foods usually resemble the way they looked in nature, other than being cut up and prepared for cooking. In contrast, refined and processed foods have been substantially altered and bear little if any resemblance to their original form. For example, a chicken breast or leg looks like part of a chicken, whereas a deep-fried chicken nugget (covered with a thick coating of flour and fried in oil) does not.

The ancient hunter-gatherer diet provided an amazing diversity of whole foods, including fish, land animals, and dozens of vegetables, collectively providing all the nutrients needed for normal gene function. For people today, eating a variety of fresh foods can approximate the ancient diet. Unfortunately, many people eat from a very narrow selection of foods, which deprives genes of their full nutritional heritage.

—ɯ—

Plan Ahead, but Keep It Simple

One of the most common nutrition problems today is not planning ahead or shopping for our next meal or two. Another difficulty is making the time to cook nutritious meals and then relax over them.

In our fast-paced society, time has become one of the scarcest of all commodities. Many of us simply do not have the time to do everything we want to do or everything others demand of us. As a consequence we often struggle to squeeze out a few extra minutes each day, such as by driving fast or eating on the go.

The irony, of course, is that we do make the time for commuting, working extra hours, and watching television but not for the mental or physical preparation of the sound nutrition that helps sustain us and maintain our health, particularly our genetic health. People often hold off eating until they are overly hungry and then they eat to quickly quench their hunger, not with the intent of obtaining good nourishment. These factors have set the stage for fast-food restaurants and even faster drive-through service, which provide almost instant but nutritionally lacking meals.

Eating more nutritiously requires a little more forethought and planning. You can do some of the mental planning during television commercials or while commuting. Keep a pad of paper and pen handy, and if you are in the car, jot down some of the specifics while waiting at a red light. Later, at the supermarket, buy the foods you will need for at least two or three meals. In terms of actual cooking, keep things simple but flavorful, with enough leftovers for a fast and tasty second meal. (Many of the recipes in chapter 8 are meant to be simple and relatively quick to prepare.) For example, you can quickly cube and stir-fry chicken with herbs and vegetables.

—ɯ—

Guideline 3: Eat Quality Protein

Fish, chicken, lean meats, eggs, and other protein-rich foods are good sources of vitamins B_6 and B_{12}, which your cells need to manufacture new DNA and repair existing DNA. In addition, the protein in these foods is broken down during digestion into its individual amino acids. These amino acids are transported from the gut to your body's individual cells, where genes provide instructions for recombining them into the specific proteins, enzymes, and other biochemicals your body needs to function.

From biological and biochemical standpoints, animal proteins are the most efficient; they are complete proteins in the sense that they contain all the nutritionally essential amino acids. Vegetarian sources of protein must be carefully combined to achieve the full suite of essential proteins. In addition, vegetarian sources of protein, such as legumes, provide substantial amounts of carbohydrate calories. In other words, legumes and other vegetarian sources of protein have less nutrient density and may be inappropriate for people who are overweight.

Specific protein sources include eggs, chicken, turkey, and lean (well-trimmed, nonmarbled) beef, pork, and lamb. In particular, protein from organically raised, free-range (grass-fed) animals is relatively low in saturated fats and high in healthy omega-3 fats, which help suppress inflammation-promoting genes. Wild game, which is also grass-fed, has levels of omega-3 fats that sometimes rival those of cold-water fish.

Corn-fed beef is often promoted as being healthy and tasty. But when farm animals are raised on corn and other grains, their levels of saturated fat increase while omega-3 concentrations virtually vanish. Keep in mind that buffalo, traditionally a type of wild game, is now often fed corn, which increases its saturated-fat levels. Whenever possible, opt for protein from grass-fed, not corn-fed, animals.

—m—

Cooking Affects Protein Quality

How you cook food affects the bioavailability of its protein and constituent amino acids.

Raw protein provides the least adulterated amino acids. Sashimi, which uses raw but high-quality cuts of fish, is usually safe when prepared by an experienced chef. Unfortunately, bacterial and parasitic contamination of meat and chicken is common and almost always requires at least some cooking.

The heat of cooking modifies the structure of proteins, and the more food is cooked—at either higher temperatures or for greater lengths of time—the greater those alterations. Heating increases the formation of advanced glycation end products (AGEs), which form from permanent bonds between sugars and proteins. AGEs can attach to and damage DNA strands, altering or disabling normal gene function. High-temperature cooking, such as grilling, generates especially large numbers of AGEs. Similarly, baking a Thanksgiving turkey for several hours also generates large numbers of AGEs in the browned skin and drier meat.

In general, faster and lighter cooking methods, such as stir-frying, are preferable because they produce fewer AGEs. Similarly, cooking in a liquid, such as poaching fish in water, limits AGE production. Thus, steaming, poaching, and rapid pan-frying and stir-frying are superior to grilling and baking. However, baking food in a broth or coating food with olive oil before baking will reduce the formation of AGEs.

—⚉—

Guideline 4: Eat a Varied Selection of Nonstarchy Vegetables

Nonstarchy vegetables include spinach, lettuces, kale, tomatoes, cucumbers, avocados, broccoli, cauliflower, green beans, and mustard greens. In particular, leafy green vegetables are rich in folic acid, a B vitamin needed for the synthesis and repair of DNA.

These vegetables are nutrient-dense because they provide large amounts of vitamins, vitamin-like phytonutrients (such as antioxidant carotenoids and flavonoids), minerals, and fiber but relatively few calories and carbohydrates. In contrast, potatoes (whether baked, mashed, or fried) are the most common starchy vegetable and are equivalent to a highly refined carbohydrate.

Nonstarchy vegetables are a treasure trove of quality nutrition. For example, broccoli contains a variety of compounds that help the liver break down toxins and prevent cancer. All told, more than six hundred antioxidant carotenoids and more than five thousand antioxidant flavonoids have been identified in plants, and many are found in vegetables.

It is worthwhile to expand your nutritional frontiers in order to obtain a wider variety of these nutrients. For example, if you have tended to eat salads with iceberg lettuce, try baby romaine lettuce and spinach. If you already eat dark-leaf lettuces and spinach, try arugula and watercress—or an assortment of mixed salad greens.

—⚉—

Discovering or Rediscovering the Joy of Cooking

Many of us, both men and women, never learned how to cook meals from scratch using fresh ingredients. In addition, today's work and home pressures often do not leave much time for cooking wholesome meals. And yet the Food Network (www.foodtv.com) remains one of the most popular networks on television. I believe that is because many people do want to cook, even if they don't always have the time.

Take heart. I didn't learn how to cook until I turned forty-nine, and now I enjoy cooking as a satisfying creative activity. Besides, cooking is the only creative activity that allows you to eat what you've made. I learned to cook by working with friends in the kitchen, watching the Food Network, reading a couple of basic cookbooks, experimenting with ingredients, and trying to make healthier versions of common meals. I paid as much attention to kitchen technique as to ingredients, just as amateur photographers pay attention to both the style and equipment of professionals. Over the past few years, I have had only a couple of culinary failures, and my friends give most of my meals high ratings.

As is the case for most people, work pressures limit my time in the kitchen. Consequently, I try to keep meals relatively simple and easy to prepare, and I also try to make efficient use of leftovers. For example, a dinner may take an investment of my precious time, but the creative use of leftovers—"planovers," as one friend calls them—saves time in preparing at least one other meal.

Make your kitchen experience a fun time. Envision yourself as an artist, with chicken, vegetables, and spices your version of an artist's palette of paints. It helps to follow recipes that are straightforward, but feel free to modify ingredients (particularly spices) to suit your tastes. If you have not done a lot of cooking, it may take you several months to become truly comfortable in the kitchen. But along the way you will gain a sense of accomplishment and confidence from the tasty meals you create.

—⚏—

Guideline 5: Eat a Varied Selection of Nonstarchy Fruits

Like nonstarchy vegetables, nonstarchy fruits provide an exceptional nutritional value for the calories they provide. Nonstarchy fruits include raspberries, blackberries, blueberries, kiwifruit, apples, melons, and grapefruit. A recent study found that kiwifruit in particular promoted the synthesis and repair of DNA.

The most common starchy fruit is the banana, but pears are also relatively high in sugars and starches. Some types of citrus, such as oranges, have been cultivated for sweetness, but occasionally eating the fruit is far better than drinking a glass of juice, which provides a lot of sugars without the fiber to buffer their absorption.

Squeezing juice from a wedge of fresh lemon or lime onto fish or poultry can add a tremendous amount of flavor, as well as a little vitamin C and antioxidant flavonoids. In addition, fruit salsas (with citrus, cantaloupe, pineapple, and cilantro) can make an excellent sauce for many types of fish, such as halibut and tilapia.

—⁓—

Easy Sauces to Dress Up Your Meals

Exceptional sauces often make for memorable meals. Unfortunately, making many sauces at home can be difficult and time-consuming.

Terrapin Ridge (www.terrapinridge.com) markets a variety of sauces that can add original flavors to chicken, pork, or beef. The company's regular sauces and so-called garnishing sauces are versatile, and most of them use quality ingredients. (As with any other food product, carefully read the list of ingredients.)

For example, Terrapin Ridge's Spicy Chipotle Squeeze Garnishing Sauce is easily adapted to a fajita sauce. (See the Chipotle Fajita recipe in chapter 8.) And despite the name, it is not overly spicy and can be used in omelettes and egg scrambles. Some of Terrapin Ridge's other sauces include Apple Dill and Rosemary, Cilantro Chili and Garlic, Apricot Honey with Tarragon, Orange Mango with Lemongrass, Roasted Yellow Pepper, and Cranberry Horseradish. Most of these sauces work well brushed over baked foods or added while stir-frying.

—⁓—

Guideline 6: Consume Only Healthy Oils and Fats

Ancient diets provided roughly the same amounts of overall fats (fatty acids) as are found in modern diets. However, the types of fat and their ratios in ancient and modern diets are vastly different.

"Fatty acids" is the umbrella scientific term for describing fats and oils. A general rule of thumb is that fats are solid and oils are liquid at room temperature, although this distinction has little to do with the actual chemical structure of individual fatty acids.

Ancient peoples consumed fats only as they naturally occurred in meat, vegetables, nuts, and seeds. They did not use pressed or refined oils, which are concentrated sources of fatty acids. Extra-virgin olive oil is the most common pressed oil, and it is literally pressed or squeezed from olives. In contrast, refined oils, which include corn, safflower, soy, and canola, are usually obtained through high-temperature chemical extraction and undergo considerably more processing.

Different types of fats turn various genes on and off and influence how cells communicate with each other. Some fats, which are deposited in cell membranes, can also accelerate the aging of cells and, in turn, your entire body. For example, many refined oils, such as corn and safflower oil, turn on genes involved in inflammation and cancer promotion. In contrast, olive oil and fish oils tend to turn off these genes, which is why they reduce the risk of disease.

Ancient peoples consumed both saturated fat and cholesterol, but the most significant change between then and now can be found in the ratio of omega-6 to omega-3 fatty polyunsaturated fatty acids. Both families of fatty acids provide the parent molecules for many of the compounds used by the body's immune system. The omega-6 family is generally proinflammatory, whereas the omega-3 family is generally antiinflammatory. In the past, dietary intake of the omega-6 and omega-3 families was relatively equal. Today people eating American (or Western) diets tend to consume about thirty times more of the proinflammatory omega-6 fatty acids. (The consequences are discussed at length in my book *The Inflammation Syndrome*.)

Your body's tissue concentrations of fatty acids generally reflect what you have consumed over months and years, and nearly all of us have grown up eating large quantities of unhealthy refined oils and trans fats. (See Guideline 12.)

To restore a more normal balance between the omega-6 and omega-3 fatty acids, you must make a concerted effort to emphasize the omega-3 family. You can do this by eating more cold-water fish (such as salmon and herring), as well as leafy green salads (which are high in linolenic acid, the parent omega-3 fat).

My first choice for cooking oil is extra-virgin olive oil, which is made from the first pressing of olives. It is high in oleic acid, a member of the related family of omega-9 fatty acids, which quells genes involved in inflammation and enhances the benefits of omega-3 fatty acids. Because olive oil flavors vary, I recommend that you try different brands.

Macadamia nut oil is my second choice for cooking oil, though it is more expensive and difficult to find. Macadamia nut oil has a slightly higher smoke point than does olive oil, so it can be used for higher-temperature cooking. Cold-pressed grapeseed oil, a pat of butter (preferably organic, from cows not injected with bovine growth hormone), and coconut oil are acceptable for occasional use.

—⋙—

The Salad Dressing Quandary

It's a common pitfall: you have just either ordered or made a healthy and nutritious salad—only to pour an unhealthy salad dressing over it.

The problem is that the vast majority of commercial salad dressings in supermarkets, fast-food places, and national chain restaurants are made with highly refined soybean or cottonseed oils, rich in omega-6 fats. Furthermore, many of these oils also contain sugars, partially hydrogenated vegetable oils, and dangerous trans fats.

You have several options. In a restaurant ask if the salad dressing is homemade (on the premises) and uses olive oil or canola oil, the latter being a reasonable compromise under the circumstances. If you cannot obtain an assurance about the oil used, then ask for simple oil and vinegar—the oil will be olive oil. (See "Ask Questions and Read the Fine Print on Labels" later in this chapter.)

At home you can make your own salad dressing, using combinations of extra-virgin olive oil, quality vinegar (such as red wine or balsamic vinegars), Italian herbs (including oregano, basil, and parsley), garlic, and lemon juice. You can also find many quality salad dressings at natural food stores, such as Wild Oats, Whole Foods, Vitamin Cottage (in Colorado and New Mexico), and the many small independent health food stores around the country. Typically, these salad dressings are made with olive oil and cold-pressed canola oil. Some of the better dressings include such brands as Stonewall Kitchen, Annie's Naturals, and Terrapin Ridge. But always read the list of ingredients carefully because some specific dressings may contain sugars or other undesirable ingredients.

—⋙—

Guideline 7: Season Your Foods with Herbs and Spices

Most people consume far too much sodium relative to potassium, reversing the ancient dietary ratio in which potassium dominated. In addition, sodium provides no nutritional value, and a sodium-potassium imbalance may be involved in a number of diseases, including edema, high blood pressure, kidney disease, and coronary heart disease.

While small amounts of RealSalt (a natural salt product) or sea salt are acceptable for most people, herbs and spices can add far more distinctive and enjoyable flavors to foods. For example, oregano and basil add a distinctly Mediterranean taste to fish, whereas dill provides a lighter, more springlike flavor. Other common culinary herbs include bay leaves, cinnamon, dill, garlic, parsley, rosemary, and thyme, and then there are blends, such as herbes de Provence.

Like vegetables and fruits, culinary herbs and spices provide a diversity of antioxidant flavonoids and related compounds. Some, such as oregano and rosemary, are especially high in antioxidants. These herbs and spices protect DNA from damage and help ensure the normal functioning of genes.

Some Acceptable High-Carb Foods in Moderation

You may occasionally wish to eat small amounts of dietary carbohydrates—for taste and satiety, for energy (if you are physically active), or for a little more variety in your diet. However, if you are overweight or suffer from insulin resistance, high fasting blood sugar, prediabetes, or diabetes, you should strictly limit your intake of carbohydrate-rich foods.

With that caveat, several carbohydrate-rich foods make excellent side dishes. Sweet potatoes and yams have a weaker effect on blood sugar and insulin levels compared with conventional potatoes, and they also have higher levels of protective antioxidant carotenoids. Both sweet potatoes and yams can be served baked and split, much the way you would prepare a baked potato. A pat of butter or a sprinkle of cinnamon enhances the flavor. You can also mash the sweet potatoes or yams.

In addition, there are many nonwhite rice varieties that can add exotic flavors to a meal. While most people are familiar with short- and long-grain brown rice, fewer have heard about red, purple, black, and green rices. Lotus Foods (www.lotusfoods.com or [510] 525-3137) markets Forbidden Rice, an exotic-tasting purple-colored rice, as well as Bhutanese Red Rice. (The name "Forbidden Rice" derives from the fact that it was once a food of Chinese royalty, which peasants were forbidden to eat.) The company's red rice flour can be used in place of regular flour for dredging fillet of sole or boneless chicken breasts. Indian Harvest (www.indianharvest.com or [800] 348-7032) markets a larger variety of rice products, including Colusari red rice, Himalayan red rice, Purple Thai rice, Chinese black rice, and Bamboo (green) rice.

—⋙—

Guideline 8: Drink Water and Teas

Thirst is the body's way of demanding greater hydration. Biologically, this is strictly a request for water, the original thirst quencher, but people now consume an astonishing array of liquids, including soft drinks, coffees, teas, breakfast drinks, and alcoholic beverages. Many of these beverages, particularly flavored coffees, contain hidden sugars.

Soft drinks, which have been called "liquid candy" by the Center for Science in the Public Interest, provide an enormous amount of refined sugars, usually in the form of high-fructose corn syrup. In fact, our consumption of sugary soft drinks has increased markedly over the years. Fifty years ago six-ounce bottles of soft drinks were the standard. Today the memory of such modest sizes is dwarfed by two-liter (sixty-four-ounce) bottles, each providing, incredibly, about one-half cup of various sugars.

The average American now consumes about 150 pounds of refined sugars each year, but such averages can be deceiving. Because my sugar consumption probably adds up to only about 5 pounds annually, someone else must make up the difference by consuming 300 pounds each year.

When you quench your thirst with a sugary soft drink, you initiate or sustain an up-and-down blood-sugar and insulin cycle that can reduce your glucose tolerance, leave you feeling tired, and impair your concentration. As you have already read, elevated insulin levels trigger a variety of changes in gene activity that increase body fat and the risk of diabetes.

When you are thirsty, it is best to do what nature really wants you to do: drink some calorie-free water, the original diet drink. If tap water doesn't excite you (either because of taste or contaminants in your community), consider using a Brita or Pūr water filter. Bottled water is also an option. You can improve the taste of filtered or bottled water by refrigerating it and by adding a wedge of lemon or lime when you serve it.

European brands of sparkling mineral water, again with a wedge of lemon or lime, make a sensible beverage with lunch or dinner. Perrier, San Pellegrino, and Gerolsteiner are among the best-known brands. They have subtle variations in flavor, resulting from differences in their mineral content. And this mineral content points to the nutritional bonus of such waters: they provide substantial amounts of calcium and magnesium.

Many herbal teas also make wonderful beverages, and Celestial Seasonings, Stash, and other companies offer a wide selection of teas that can be brewed hot or cold. You can make a "sun tea" by allowing several tea bags to steep in a pitcher of water either out in the sun or on your kitchen counter. One of my favorite sun teas is Celestial Seasonings Red Zinger. Black tea, green tea, and white tea are other options, and while they contain some caffeine, they are also rich in antioxidant flavonoids, and their health benefits seem to override any caffeine-related health problems. These teas appear to lower the long-term risk of cardiovascular diseases and cancer.

When it comes to coffee, the research is nothing less than conflicting and confusing. Modest amounts of coffee—two cups or less daily—do not appear to pose health problems for many people. However, drinking larger quantities—five to ten cups daily—can make people feel edgy, irritable, and impatient. Also, coffee does not contain the antioxidant flavonoids found in teas. If you like your coffee and don't want to give it up, consider drinking two cups or fewer daily, unsweetened, and organically grown.

—⚏—

Snacks and Desserts

Many people have a nearly insatiable sweet tooth. But your sensitivity to sweet foods reveals a lot about your glucose tolerance.

As your glucose tolerance decreases—that is, as your blood-sugar and insulin levels lean more toward diabetes—you become less sensitive to the taste of sweets. This means you need more sugar to make a food or drink taste sweet to you. As a general rule of thumb, a person who uses three teaspoons of sugar in a cup of coffee has poorer glucose tolerance than a person who uses one or none.

When you limit your intake of sugars and refined carbohydrates, you can greatly improve your glucose tolerance—and the genetic impairments and damage that usually accompany elevated blood-sugar and insulin levels. As your diet and glucose tolerance improve, nuts and nut butters will taste sweeter and will more likely satisfy your sweet tooth.

You can make your own trail nut mixes with unsalted cashews, pistachios, peanuts, almonds, filberts, pumpkin seeds, and (preferably organic) raisins. Other options include a little peanut or almond butter on apple or banana slices, or a small amount of honey drizzled on Greek yogurt, available at many specialty food stores. (See the recipe in chapter 8.)

However, if you are trying to lose weight or if you have serious glucose tolerance problems (such as prediabetes or diabetes), it is best for you to avoid any sugary dessert, snack, or beverage.

—⁊⁊—

Guideline 9: Eat Organically Produced Foods Whenever Possible

Foods grown with organic (or sustainable) agricultural methods avoid the use of synthetic fertilizers and pesticides. Such techniques enhance rather than reduce soil quality, which is good for both you and the environment. You benefit from higher levels of nutrients and fewer contaminants in foods, and the environment benefits from less pesticide, hormone, and antibiotic runoff.

Many people will say that organic fruits and vegetables taste better than conventional produce. It could be that they do in fact taste better, or it could be that they are simply delivered to markets faster and fresher. Most commercial, nonorganic tomatoes are picked green (so they are less likely to bruise during shipping) and sprayed with ethylene gas to turn them red. Unfortunately, they still taste like green tomatoes. In contrast, organically raised tomatoes are often vine-ripened and taste the way commercial tomatoes did forty years ago.

Better taste is only one of the benefits of organic foods. Several studies have found that organically raised fruits and vegetables have higher levels of vitamin C and antioxidant flavonoids compared with conventionally grown produce. In other words, the nutritional value of organic foods is greater than that of most commercial produce, which is grown with synthetic fertilizers and pesticides. The reason for the higher nutritional value is fascinating: plants increase their production of antioxidant flavonoids when stressed by bad weather or insects, and some flavonoids function as natural insecticides (though they are not harmful to people). Pesticides kill insects, so plants grow relatively unstressed—and with lower levels of flavonoids.

There are other compelling reasons to minimize your intake of pesticides. The most widely used pesticides function as estrogen mimics, meaning that they simulate the effects of estrogen in the body. And it's not just the pesticides used in the growing of fruits and vegetables. Even the grains fed to livestock are commonly laced with pesticides to prevent insect infestation. In some animal species exposed to pesticide runoff in rivers and lakes, male sexual organs do not fully develop, indicating a fundamental alteration of gene behavior. No scientific studies have shown that this happens in people, but it has been shown that children eating conventionally grown produce do consume large amounts of pesticides along with it.

Similarly, chicken and meat from organically raised or free-range animals will likely be free of pesticides and added hormones. The same is true for dairy products. Organic milk, cream, and butter are obtained from cows that have not been injected with bovine growth hormone to stimulate milk production.

The principal drawbacks to organic foods are availability and price, although many supermarkets now contain a small selection of organic produce. Still, organically produced foods often cost 10 to 20 percent more than conventional foods. The higher price is related to economies of scale. Organic foods are usually the result of small-scale farming activities, whereas conventional foods are grown using more efficient, large-scale methods. As interest in organic foods increases, and the numbers and sizes of organic farms increase as a result, pricing will likely become more competitive. So for now, if you can purchase organic foods, do so. But you can follow most of the dietary guidelines in this book with conventionally grown foods.

—⟋⟍—

Ask Questions and Read the Fine Print on Labels

A few years ago, when blood tests showed that my iron was elevated (a risk factor for heart disease), a nutritionist suggested that I avoid breads and pastas. Puzzled, I asked why. She explained that these foods were fortified with iron, which I did not need. When I looked at the fine print of food labels, I discovered that she was right. I'd had no idea that iron was added to these foods.

Most food ingredients must, by federal law, be listed on packages. I say "most" because food processors sometimes play a shell game to avoid listing certain ingredients. For example, "natural flavors" is a vague statement that could refer to culinary herbs, sugars, or monosodium glutamate (MSG, a flavor enhancer that makes some people ill).

It is important that you not be influenced by pleasant-sounding but promotional words, such as "natural," "organic," or "low-carb" on the front of a package. Instead it is to your benefit to become a compulsive reader of the fine print on the back or sides of food packages. It is here that you will find a list of ingredients in order of their weight. It is best to avoid unhealthy oils (such as partially hydrogenated vegetable oils), various forms of sugar (such as sucrose, glucose, fructose, high-fructose corn syrup, and dextrose), wheat gluten, artificial colorings, stabilizers, and chemicals added to make the manufacturing process easier.

The term "organic" may also be misused. Several years ago a leading cereal maker marketed a 100 percent organic cereal. The problem was that most of the ingredients were refined grains and sugars, so despite being organic, the cereal was not any better nutritionally than a nonorganic product.

In restaurants it is important to inquire politely about food ingredients in various meals. I happen to be allergic to tomato, so I often ask whether tomato—in any form—might be used. Sometimes tomato powder or dried tomato pieces are used in recipes, and occasionally finely diced tomato is sprinkled on top of a meal as a garnish. I know some people who are sensitive to gluten, so they always ask that fish not be dredged in flour. Most restaurants want to accommodate their customers, and most waiters and waitresses are willing to check with the chef and have a meal modified to satisfy a customer. For example, for a quick lunch out, I will often order a grilled chicken breast or a turkey burger, but without the bun and with vegetables (preferably steamed) instead of fries. I have not yet been refused this accommodation.

However, don't expect this type of customer service at fast-food restaurants and lower-quality national chain restaurants. Like military kitchens, they are geared toward high-volume food preparation and don't gladly make exceptions. That's because much of the food in these restaurants arrives either frozen or prepackaged, ready to heat and serve.

—ᴍ—

Guideline 10: Restrict or Avoid Refined Carbohydrates and Sugars, and Limit Your Intake of All Processed Carbohydrates

Refined carbohydrates and sugars offer the opposite of a nutrient-dense diet: they contain plenty of calories that are almost devoid of other nutritional value. They displace more nutritious foods, such as protein sources and vegetables. Furthermore, their consumption elevates levels of the hormone insulin, which in turn activates genes involved in promoting obesity, inflammation, diabetes, and heart disease.

Most refined carbohydrates fall into two groups: sugars and grain-derived food products. The two most common sugars are sucrose (table sugar) and high-fructose corn syrup. They are almost omnipresent in processed foods, with sugar added to salt and even to so-called sugar substitutes, such as Sweet'n Low and Equal. Refined carbohydrate starches are created through the processing of grains, such as wheat, corn, or rice, and are most commonly found in flour, breads, pastas, croutons, bakery confections, and breakfast bars. Nearly all processed and manufactured foods—those that come in boxes at the supermarket—contain various blends of sugars, grain-based refined carbohydrates, and highly refined oils.

And what of whole-wheat or whole-grain breads, among the icons of natural foods? In many respects whole grains are healthier than white. However, even the best whole-grain products have been heavily processed and provide mostly carbohydrate calories. This view is virtual heresy in the health food industry, but the fact is that human teeth cannot chew raw grains. In order to be made edible, grains must be ground (processed), which increases their available carbohydrates and reduces their fiber (a carbohydrate blocker).

Yet another problem is that many grains, including wheat, rye, and barley, contain gluten, a highly allergenic protein and the cause of celiac disease. Approximately one in a hundred people are genetically sensitive to gluten, although some researchers have suggested that as many as one in two have some degree of gluten sensitivity.

White or so-called red potatoes, whether baked, mashed, or fried, have an effect on blood-sugar and insulin levels that is almost indistinguishable from that of a soft drink and a doughnut. The same is true with white rice. Ironically, many overweight people diet and snack on rice cakes, which rapidly boost blood-sugar and insulin levels—and actually contribute to weight gain and diabetes risk. Other options—in moderation—include sweet potatoes, yams, and various types of brown, red, purple, and black rices. (See "Some Acceptable High-Carb Foods in Moderation" earlier in this chapter.)

—⁓—

Do Heated Carbs Create Carcinogens?

In 2000, Swedish researchers garnered headlines after reporting that large amounts of a known cancer-causing substance, acrylamide, were found in french fries, breakfast cereals, crackers, and many other foods. Not unexpectedly, representatives of processed-food companies reacted skeptically, and the U.S. Food and Drug Administration took essentially no action at all.

Since then additional research has confirmed the formation of acrylamide, an ingredient in many plastics, in carbohydrate-rich foods cooked at high temperatures. Scientists have also figured out the mystery of how it forms. Acrylamide is similar to the amino acid asparagine, which is found in many carbohydrate-containing foods. When asparagine is heated to very high temperatures, such as during frying or high-temperature baking and processing, it converts to acrylamide.

French fries can contain up to almost 3,000 mcg of acrylamide per kilogram (2.2 pounds). While no one knows the amount of acrylamide that will actually increase a person's risk of cancer, exposure to acrylamide undoubtedly adds to the many carcinogens already present in our foods and our environment—and to our risk of developing cancer.

All in all, the acrylamide story may be another reminder that people were not meant to eat highly processed carbohydrates, and that we should eat more wholesome foods.

—⁓—

Guideline 11: Minimize Your Consumption of Highly Refined Cooking Oils

Highly refined cooking oils, including corn, safflower, soybean, and cottonseed oils, are commonly used in processed foods. People did not consume these oils until relatively recently, and they have many undesirable health effects. You should do your best to avoid them, and following this guideline requires that you carefully read food labels. (Olive oil, as previously discussed, does not fall into this group.)

These cooking oils are rich in linoleic acid, the parent molecule of omega-6 fats. Because of the preponderance of refined and processed foods, most people now consume excessive amounts of omega-6 fats. As a result, omega-6 fats have largely displaced dietary omega-3 fats, found in fish, grass-fed animal protein, and leafy green vegetables. In general, omega-6 fats help turn on genes involved in chronic inflammation, which is intertwined with the aging process and most degenerative diseases.

The problem is more serious than just the sheer quantity of omega-6 fats in the modern diet. When heated (cooked), the omega-6 fats generate large amounts of harmful free radicals. If you eat a piece of fried chicken and some fried potatoes, you consume these free-radical-oxidized fats, which are subsequently incorporated into your body's cells. These oxidized fats generate still more free radicals—think of them as part of a biological domino theory—which in turn damage DNA, interfere with normal gene activity, and prematurely age non-DNA cell structures. For example, normal cell membranes, which consist largely of different types of fats, are flexible and serve as passageways for nutrients entering and waste products leaving cells. Free-radical oxidation essentially seals these passageways, blocking the entry of needed nutrients and preventing the exit of waste materials. In effect, such free-radical damage prevents the restocking of a cell's kitchen and the flushing of its toilet.

The genetic implications of excessive consumption of omega-6 fats are frightening. Research has shown that omega-6-rich corn and safflower oils are potent promoters of cancer-cell growth. Perhaps not surprisingly, the omega-3 fats have cancer-inhibiting effects. Both families of fats influence the genetic programming of cancer cells, but in opposite ways.

For years polyunsaturated fats have been recommended for reducing the risk of coronary heart disease. Unfortunately, public health authorities have rarely distinguished between the omega-6 and omega-3 fats. As it turns out, the omega-6 fats seem to increase the risk of heart disease and age-related macular degeneration, the leading cause of blindness among the elderly. In contrast, considerable research indicates that the omega-3 fats protect against these diseases.

As a general rule, follow Guideline 6, which recommends extra-virgin olive oil for most of your cooking. When eating out, avoid fast-food and national chain restaurants, which typically use large amounts of omega-6 fats. Don't eat fried foods, such as fried chicken and french fries. Instead opt for restaurants serving Italian, Greek, Middle Eastern, or "new American" cuisine, or other restaurants that, as a general rule, use olive oil in cooking.

Guideline 12: Avoid All Foods with Partially Hydrogenated Vegetable Oils and Trans Fats

Along with sugars, refined carbohydrates, and highly refined omega-6 fatty acids, partially hydrogenated vegetable oils are one of the most common ingredients in modern processed foods. This particular type of vegetable oil is found in many margarines, salad dressings, vegetable shortening, breads, cookies, muffins, and literally thousands of prepackaged convenience foods, as well as in many fast foods.

Partially hydrogenated vegetable oils are manufactured by adding hydrogen atoms to vegetable oils, such as soybean oil, and they are rich in trans-fatty acids. Hydrogenation increases the manufacturability and shelf life of oils, but it has serious health consequences.

Trans-fatty acids are rare in nature, and numerous studies have found that they increase the risk of developing cardiovascular diseases far more than do saturated fats. Is there a safe amount of trans-fatty acids? Many experts say there is not.

As I wrote in *The Inflammation Syndrome*, trans-fatty acids interfere with the enzymes involved in processing the omega-6 and omega-3 families of fatty acids. As a consequence they literally gum up the body's processing of these two important groups of fats. It is very likely also that trans-fatty acids do much of their dirty work by altering the expression of genes involved in fat metabolism. One recent study found that diets high in trans-fatty acids increased the formation of small particles of low-density lipoprotein (LDL), which are more likely to promote heart disease than are the larger LDL particles.

If there is one food product you should never make an exception in avoiding, it is trans-fatty acids. But avoiding them is currently easier said than done. They are in nearly all fried, boxed, and baked foods. As an example, many brands of breakfast bars, advertised as a nutritious "breakfast on the run" for busy people, contain large amounts of trans-fatty acids. In some breakfast bars, half of the fat is identified as saturated, which is odd for a nonanimal product—until you realize that the saturated-fat levels represent trans-fatty acids.

The Food and Drug Administration has ruled that food companies must start listing the quantity of trans-fatty acids on food labels, but companies will not be required to do so until January 2006.

In sum, these dietary guidelines emphasize nutrient-dense foods such as fish, chicken, and nonstarchy vegetables over nutrient-poor sugars, carbohydrates, and unhealthy fats. By following these dietary guidelines, you will foster a cellular environment that helps your genes to function at their best. In the next chapter, you will find a "food palette" containing many of the acceptable foods and a variety of recipes.

8

Recipes, Menu Plans, and Guidelines for Eating Out

The dietary guidelines in the previous chapter provide the nutritional framework for feeding your genes right. Here we put these guidelines into practice with recipes, menu plans, and guidelines for selecting restaurants and eating out.

Over the past century, our society has changed from one in which nearly all meals were home-cooked from fresh ingredients to one in which only one-third of meals are homemade. Hand in hand with this shift in eating habits has come a change in cooking habits. Fewer people know how to cook a meal with fresh ingredients, and a recent survey found that only about half of home meals even involved turning on the stove!

If cooking seems like an ancient or dying art, it remains one that is surprisingly easy to learn or relearn. However, if the prospect of cooking a meal makes you nervous, there are several ways to increase your comfort level. First, watch the Food Network on television, paying as much attention to the preparation and cooking techniques of chefs as to the foods they use. Second, browse cookbooks and cooking magazines, paying particular attention to easy-to-prepare meals. Finally, check your area's resources for introductory cooking classes, which may be offered by community colleges or stores that sell kitchen tools.

When you are ready to cook some meals from scratch—that is, avoiding anything that comes in a box or can—here's how to proceed:

- Plan your major meals, such as dinner, a day or two in advance. Decide on a recipe, and make a shopping list so you buy all the ingredients you will need. For now stick with ingredients you are familiar with, and avoid the exotic.
- Keep your initial meals simple, straightforward, and uncomplicated. They will be easier and faster to prepare. Stir-fried meals are a great way to start.
- Don't rush. If your favorite television show is about to come on, set up your VCR to tape it. Take your time, and enjoy cutting up vegetables and, let's say, a piece of boneless and skinless chicken breast. Cooking can be a fun, creative, and sensual experience, so approach it with a positive attitude.
- Make enough food to have some leftovers. You can use them for breakfast, lunch, or dinner the next day, and that will save you time. When you start with quality ingredients, your leftovers will taste surprisingly good.
- Experiment with quantities, particularly of herbs. I enjoy their rich flavor and usually add far more than most recipes call for. Most of the recipes in this book allow for a great deal of flexibility in terms of the amounts of ingredients.

Use a Food Palette

It may help you to follow and personalize what I call a "food palette." Artists use a palette to dab and mix colors of paints before applying them to a canvas, and the *Feed Your Genes Right* food palette has a similar function: it provides an assortment of foods, divided into different groups, that you can combine in the kitchen. In a sense this food palette is good for your palate!

The *Feed Your Genes Right* Food Palette

The rationale behind this food palette, which you can expand upon, is that it provides a selection of nutrient-dense foods, which foster healthy DNA and normal gene function. Collectively, these foods are rich sources of protein, vitamins, minerals, fiber, and healthy fats, but they contain only small amounts of carbohydrates. Legumes are listed under starchy foods, not protein sources, because they contain a substantial amount of carbohydrate relative to their protein. The food palette does not include refined sugars and refined carbohydrates, which trigger abnormal genetic responses leading to obesity, diabetes, and Syndrome X.

Protein Sources

These protein sources provide both amino acids and vitamins. Select one serving from this group as part of your meal:

chicken (various cuts)	game meats (various cuts)
eggs	shellfish
fish	turkey (various cuts)

Optional protein sources include these:

beef (lean)	lamb	yogurt (unsweetened or sugar-free)
hard cheeses	pork	

Vegetables for Cooking

Vegetables are high in vitamins, minerals, healthy fats, and fiber. Select one, two, or three vegetables from this group each day:

broccoli	green beans	onions
carrots	kale	shallots
cauliflower	leek	spinach
fennel (anise) bulbs	mushrooms	
garlic	mustard greens	

Vegetables for Salads

These vegetables, served cold, are also high in vitamins, minerals, healthy fats, and fiber. Select one, two, or three vegetables from this group each day:

arugula	lettuces, such as Boston lettuce or romaine	tomatoes
cucumber	radicchio	watercress
endive	spinach	

Fruits

These fruits are high in vitamins, minerals, healthy fats, and fiber. Select one, two, or three fruits from this group, as a side dish each day with breakfast or as dessert after lunch and/or dinner:

apples	grapefruit	strawberries
blackberries	honeydew	watermelon
blueberries	kiwifruit	
cantaloupe	raspberries	

Starchy Foods

Select one of these, but in a small amount:

brown, red, purple, black, and green rice (not white!)	yam
wild rice (a grass, not a rice)	legumes
sweet potato	

Cooking Oils and Fats

Select one of these, but use it sparingly:

extra-virgin olive oil	macadamia nut oil	butter

Seasonings

Select one or two of these, based on recipes and personal tastes:

basil	herbes de Provence	thyme
bay leaves	oregano	saffron
cayenne	parsley	garlic
cinnamon	rosemary	
dill	sage	

Nonherb Seasonings

Although most people do not consider citrus juices to be seasonings, small amounts of one of these can brighten the flavors of fish, shellfish, chicken, and turkey:

lemon juice	lime juice

Choose one of these optional seasonings that may be used occasionally and sparingly with (but not in place of) the above herbs:

fresh-ground pepper	sea salt or RealSalt

Beverages

Select one of these for each meal:

water: filtered tap or bottled	herbal tea (many varieties)
sparkling mineral water	wine (in moderation)
tea: black, green, or white	

Cooking Methods

Use one of these cooking methods to prepare the previously mentioned foods (except for salads and fruit). Note that some foods will not lend themselves to all methods of preparation.

sautéing	pan frying
stir frying	baking (preferably under thirty minutes)
poaching	boiling
steaming	

Dinner Main Courses

Chipotle Fajitas   (Serves 2–3)

1 pat of butter
1 tablespoon either macadamia nut oil or extra-virgin olive oil
1 medium yellow or red onion, sliced
1 large or 2 small red bell peppers, cored and cut into strips
2 tablespoons Terrapin Ridge Spicy Chipotle Squeeze Garnishing Sauce (see chapter 7, or go www.terrapinridge.com)

1 pound boneless, skinless chicken breasts, sliced into 3-inch strips
4 low-carb whole-wheat tortillas
sour cream (organic preferred)
grated cheddar cheese (organic preferred)

Heat the butter and oil on medium heat in a wok or a skillet. Sauté the onion and bell peppers. Add 1 tablespoon of chipotle sauce. When the onion and peppers are soft, after about 5 to 10 minutes, add the chicken and stir-fry. After the chicken starts to turn white, add 1 to 2 more teaspoons of chipotle sauce and continue to stir-fry. (The chipotle sauce is not exceptionally hot, so you can adjust the amount to suit your personal tastes.) When cooked, reduce the heat to a simmer. Heat the tortillas in a microwave, about 20 seconds, on medium setting. Serve the fajitas in the center of the tortillas, adding sour cream and cheese at the table. Alternative preparation: use either shrimp or steak slices instead of chicken.

Salmon with Coconut Milk Sauce   (Serves 2)

2 salmon fillets, about ⅓ to ½ pound each	3 shiitake mushrooms, diced
olive oil	½ teaspoon coriander
1 pat of butter	1½ cups coconut milk
1 large or 2 medium shallots, diced	1 tablespoon coconut flakes
	juice of 1 lime

Preparing the fish: Lightly coat the salmon fillets with olive oil and bake at 350 degrees, about 8 to 10 minutes per inch of thickness.

For the sauce: Melt the butter on medium heat in an 8-inch skillet. Add the shallots and sauté. When the shallots are soft, add the mushrooms. When the mushrooms are soft, sprinkle on the coriander and stir. Add the coconut milk and continue stirring. Turn the heat down to low. Add the coconut flakes and lime juice. Stir the cream sauce to prevent it from thickening. The total cooking time for the sauce is about 10 to 12 minutes.

To serve: Transfer the salmon to a plate and pour the sauce over the fish. Alternatively, flake the salmon into a bowl, add the sauce, and gently mix, creating more of a stew texture. Serve with vegetables and brown rice.

Simple Trout Amandine   (Serves 2)

1–2 tablespoons extra-virgin olive oil	2 tablespoons sliced raw almonds
1–2 tablespoons butter	¼ teaspoon dried dill or parsley
2 trout fillets, about ⅓ pound each	juice of 1–2 limes
Lotus brand Bhutanese red rice flour	pinch each of salt and pepper

Heat the olive oil and butter on medium heat in a 12-inch skillet. Meanwhile, rinse the trout fillets, pat them with a paper towel to remove excess water, and dredge them in the red rice flour (available at www.lotusfoods.com). Do not try to remove the skin from the bottom of the fillet; the fish will easily pull from the skin after it is cooked. Place the fillets skin sides up in the skillet and cook for 3 minutes; then turn them over and cook for another 2 to 3 minutes. Remove the fillets from the skillet to a platter, but do not pour off the butter and olive oil. Add the almonds and sauté, then add the dill or parsley and lime juice, along with salt and pepper. Cook the almonds for 1 to 2 minutes and then pour them over the fillets. The amandine sauce can also be poured over accompanying brown rice and steamed vegetables.

Chicken with Mustard Sauce (Serves 2–3)

2 tablespoons Terrapin Ridge
  Cracked Pepper, Lemon and
  Thyme Mustard (see chapter 7)*
2 tablespoons water
1–1½ pounds boneless, skinless
  chicken breast, cubed

1 tablespoon extra-virgin olive oil
1 pat of butter
1 tablespoon capers
juice of 1 lemon

Mix the mustard with the water so that the texture is smooth, not lumpy. Meanwhile, cube the chicken into approximately ½- to 1-inch pieces. Heat the olive oil and butter on medium heat in a large skillet or wok. Add the chicken and stir-fry the cubed pieces until they are mostly cooked. Add the mustard sauce and then the capers, and continue stir-frying so that the chicken cubes turn yellow. Turn down the heat and simmer until the chicken is cooked.

*Available from www. terrapinridge.com. Alternatively, you can start with a Dijon mustard, freshly ground pepper, and lemon juice.

Scallops with Saffron Sauce (Serves 3)

1½ cups fish stock
1 tablespoon dry vermouth
¼–½ teaspoon ground saffron
¼ to ½ pint whipping cream
4 ounces fresh baby spinach leaves

12 sea scallops (large)
2 pats of butter
1 teaspoon olive oil
salt and pepper to taste

This meal is more complicated to prepare than others in this book and is best done by two people working together in the kitchen.

For the sauce: Bring the fish stock† to a boil in a saucepan and then simmer and reduce to thicken, about 30 to 50 minutes. While simmering, add the vermouth and saffron and stir. About 20 minutes before serving, add the heavy cream and stir. At this point estimate the amount of sauce you will need and transfer the rest to a container that can be refrigerated for several days. If you wish to thicken the sauce, prepare arrowroot thickener and stir into the sauce, but serve within 10 minutes of thickening. (See the sidebar on using arrowroot, following this recipe.)

For the spinach: Boil water in a 2-quart saucepan. Meanwhile, pinch the stems off the spinach leaves and place the leaves in a colander in the sink. When the water boils, pour it over the spinach to wilt it. Place a layer of spinach on part of a dinner plate.

For the scallops: Rinse the scallops, remove the muscle from each one, and pat them dry. Heat the butter and olive oil in a large nonstick skillet. Carefully place the scallops in the pan and cook them on medium heat for about 4 minutes; then turn them over and cook for another 4 minutes. Sprinkle with salt and pepper. Cut one scallop open to test that they are done but not overcooked. Using tongs, place the shallots on top of the spinach. To serve, drizzle the sauce over the scallops.

†You may use a commercially prepared fish stock, such as Perfect Addition Rich Fish Stock, which can be found in the freezer section of many natural food stores and supermarkets.

—∞—

Arrowroot as a Sauce Thickener

In many respects arrowroot is superior to other thickeners, such as cornstarch, because allergic sensitivities to it are rare. Arrowroot powder has a neutral flavor and delicately thickens sauces. However, the sauce cannot be boiled, and it must be used within 10 minutes of thickening. (Sauces thickened with arrowroot will not hold longer than 10 minutes, and they do not reheat well.)

Plan to use about 2½ teaspoons of arrowroot for each cup of finished sauce. To prepare arrowroot, mix it with approximately the same amount of water in a small bowl and stir rapidly with a fork or small whisk. Add very small amounts as necessary to achieve a thick paste-like texture. Next add this paste to the heated sauce (as in the above recipe) and stir or whisk rapidly. Serve within 10 minutes.

—∞—

Seafood and Rice (Serves 4–5)

1 cup short-grain brown rice	4–6 garlic cloves, diced
1 cup chicken broth*	1 large scallion, diced
1 cup water	1 teaspoon dried oregano
8 medium to large shrimp, cut into small pieces	1 teaspoon dried basil
10 small scallops, cut in half	2 tablespoons chopped fresh basil
2 tablespoons olive oil	juice of 1 lemon and 1 lime, combined
2 shallots, peeled and diced	salt to taste

Cook the rice in a saucepan with the chicken broth and water. Bring the rice to a boil and then simmer it for about 40 minutes, or until the broth boils away. While the rice is cooking, cut the shrimp and the scallops into ¼- to ½-inch pieces. In a wok or skillet, heat the olive oil and sauté the shallots, garlic, and scallion. When they are soft, add the shrimp and scallop pieces. Next add the oregano and dried basil. Sauté for approximately 2 to 3 minutes, until the shrimp turn pink and firm. Add the fresh basil at the very end. Transfer the rice to a glass bowl and add the seafood sauté. Mix thoroughly, add the lemon and lime juice, then the salt, and serve.

*Use Health Valley, Pacific, or other high-quality brand or chicken broth.

Shrimp with Artichoke Hearts and Dijon Sauce   (Serves 3–4)

2 tablespoons Dijon mustard
1 tablespoon water
2 tablespoons olive oil
4 garlic cloves, diced
6 artichoke hearts, sliced in quarters

1 pound peeled and deveined
  shrimp
juice of 1 lemon
½ teaspoon freshly ground pepper,
  or to taste

Prepare the sauce by mixing the Dijon mustard with the water in a small bowl. Meanwhile, heat the olive oil over medium heat in a non-stick wok or skillet. Sauté the garlic for about a minute. Add the artichoke hearts and sauté for another minute, then add the shrimp and sauté until they turn pink. Add the mustard sauce, continue sautéing, and then add the lemon juice. Add the freshly ground pepper and serve.

Shrimp Marinated with Garlic and Shallots   (Serves 2–4)

10 garlic cloves, diced
2 shallots, diced
1 teaspoon dried basil
1 teaspoon dried oregano
1 tablespoon fresh parsley leaves,
  chopped

2 tablespoons extra-virgin olive oil
juice of 2 limes
1 pound shrimp, peeled and
  deveined
Romano cheese, shredded
freshly ground black pepper, to taste

The rich, flavorful marinade will be cooked with the shrimp, so it should be relatively thick in consistency. In a large bowl, mix together the garlic, shallots, basil, oregano, and parsley. Next add enough of the olive oil and lime juice to create a thick (not watery) marinade. Be sure to mix the ingredients thoroughly. Add the shrimp and rub them with the marinade. Cover and refrigerate for 1 to 3 hours. (The marinade may turn the shrimp white, which is normal.) When you're ready to cook, heat a large skillet over medium heat and add the shrimp and the marinade. Sauté the shrimp until they turn pink. Sprinkle some shredded (not grated) Romano cheese over the shrimp, allow to melt slightly (about 30 seconds), then serve. Add a little freshly ground pepper, to taste.

Fillet of Sole with Almonds and Parsley   (Serves 3–4)

2 tablespoons sliced almonds
⅔–1 pound fillet of sole
¼ cup Lotus Foods Bhutanese Red Rice flour or other rice flour
1–2 tablespoons extra-virgin olive oil

1–2 pats of butter (optional)
¼ cup chopped fresh Italian (flat) parsley leaves
juice of 1 lemon

Toast the almonds in a nonstick skillet, occasionally stirring them, for about 2 minutes. Remove the almonds from the skillet and temporarily transfer them to a small plate or bowl. Rinse and pat dry the sole and dredge each piece in the red rice flour. Heat the olive oil and butter in the skillet over medium heat. Add the sole and cook for a maximum of 1 to 2 minutes per side. As the second side is cooking, sprinkle on the almonds and parsley, followed by the lemon juice. Serve immediately.

Baked Turkey Scaloppine Piccata   (Serves 4)

1½ pounds turkey tenderloin, membrane removed, sliced into pieces about the size of a silver dollar
about 1 cup high-quality chicken broth*
2 tablespoons extra-virgin olive oil
juice of 1 lemon

juice of 2 limes
10 garlic cloves, diced
2 shallots, diced
1 teaspoon coriander
2 teaspoons dried oregano
1–2 tablespoons small capers

Lay the turkey pieces in a medium baking dish. Add the chicken broth so that it covers the turkey. Next disperse the olive oil and lemon and lime juices as evenly as possible. Add the garlic, shallots, coriander, oregano, and capers. Bake for approximately 20 minutes at 350 degrees.

*Use Health Valley, Pacific, or other high-quality brand of chicken broth.

Chicken and Chanterelle Mushrooms in Cream Sauce   (Serves 4)

3 tablespoons butter
1 tablespoon extra-virgin olive oil
6 garlic cloves, diced
2 large shallots, diced
¼–½ cup chanterelle mushrooms

2 tablespoons pine nuts
1½ teaspoons dried basil
1½ teaspoons dried oregano
1–1½ pounds chicken, cubed
2–3 tablespoons whipping cream

Melt the butter in a skillet over medium heat. Add the olive oil and heat it; then sauté the garlic and shallots. Add the mushrooms, pine nuts, basil, and oregano. Cover the skillet (foil will suffice if a lid is not available) whenever you are not stirring or adding ingredients. Add the chicken and sauté. When the chicken appears cooked, add the whipping cream and stir. Add more basil and oregano, if desired, and stir before serving.

Roasted Chicken with Rosemary and Garlic   (Serves 4)

1 chicken, a 4–5-pound free-range
   fryer

8 garlic cloves, minced
2 teaspoons minced fresh rosemary

Preheat the oven to 400 degrees. Remove and dispose of the giblets. Then rinse the chicken inside and out, and pat it dry with a paper towel. Place it breast-side up in a roasting pan. With your fingers gently separate the skin from the breast and rub the garlic and rosemary on and underneath the skin. Rub any extra garlic and rosemary inside the cavity. Place the pan in the center of the preheated oven. Roast approximately 1 hour for the first 4 pounds, 7 to 8 minutes for each additional pound. The chicken will be cooked when a meat thermometer, inserted into a breast, registers 170 degrees. Remove the chicken from the oven, cover it with foil, and let it stand for 10 minutes before serving.

You can use any leftovers in Chicken and Egg Salad (page 131).

Side Dishes

Sautéed Spinach and Shiitake Mushrooms   (Serves 2)

3 tablespoons extra-virgin olive oil
4 garlic cloves, diced
3 shiitake mushrooms, rinsed, patted
   dry, and sliced
3 tablespoons pine nuts

12 ounces spinach leaves, cleaned,
   stems removed
1–2 tablespoons shredded (not
   grated) Romano cheese

Heat the olive oil in a wok. Sauté the garlic, mushrooms, and pine nuts until they are soft. Add the spinach and sauté until it is wilted. Turn off the heat and sprinkle on the cheese. Serve.

Sautéed Mushrooms and Romano Cheese   (Serves 3–4)

1 teaspoon extra-virgin olive oil
½ cup sliced white mushrooms
¼ cup sliced shiitake mushrooms
¼ cup sliced chanterelle mushrooms

½ teaspoon garlic powder
2 tablespoons shredded (not grated) Romano cheese

Heat the olive oil in a nonstick skillet over medium heat. Add all the mushrooms and sauté them until they soften, about 5 minutes. Add the garlic powder while sautéing. Reduce the heat and sprinkle the Romano cheese over the mushrooms. The mushrooms are ready to serve when the cheese is partially melted.

Roasted Carrots and Shallots*   (Serves 4)

5 large carrots, cut into ½- to 1-inch pieces
6–8 shallots, peeled and cut in half
1 tablespoon plus 1–2 teaspoons extra-virgin olive oil

1 tablespoon coarse (whole-grain) mustard
1 teaspoon honey
seasoning salt/herb mix to taste
salt and pepper to taste

Preheat the oven to 350 degrees. Spread the carrots and shallots in a baking dish and add about ¼ to ½ inch of water and 1 tablespoon of extra-virgin olive oil. Mix to coat the carrots and shallots and bake for approximately 50 minutes. Stir periodically so the vegetables do not dry or burn. After the baking is done, heat 1 to 2 teaspoons of the olive oil in a large skillet. Using a slotted spoon, transfer the carrots and shallots to this skillet and sauté. (Discard the oil and water mixture from the baking dish.) Add the mustard, honey, and seasoning, including salt and pepper, to taste. Continue to sauté, stirring periodically, for about 10 minutes until the carrots are soft (but not mushy).

*Adapted from Feast, Tucson, Arizona (www.eatatfeast.com)

Sautéed Fennel, Olives, and Raisins*   (Serves 4)

2 fennel bulbs
1 tablespoon extra-virgin olive oil
2 tablespoons diced black olives (Kalamata preferred)

2 tablespoons organic Thompson raisins
juice of 1 lemon

Remove and discard all stems from the fennel bulbs. Slice the bulbs into strips, none wider than a soda straw. Heat the olive oil in a large nonstick skillet or wok. Sauté the fennel strips, stirring every 10 minutes or so, until they are tender and start to caramelize, for possibly as long as 1 hour. (Use this time to prepare an entrée, such as Chicken with Mustard Sauce on page 123, to go with this side dish.) When the fennel is cooked, add the olives and raisins and reduce the heat to a simmer, stirring to mix the ingredients. Add the lemon juice, stir, and serve.

*Adapted from Feast, Tucson, Arizona (www.eatatfeast.com)

Simple Baked Asparagus   (Serves 3)

12 ounces fresh asparagus

¼ medium red onion, thinly sliced into rings

extra-virgin olive oil

1 tablespoon chopped fresh oregano

Preheat the oven to 400 degrees. Cut off about 1 inch of the woody bottoms of the asparagus stems. Then use a vegetable peeler to remove the skin along the lower part of the stem. Lay the asparagus spears on a baking sheet. Arrange the onion rings on top of the asparagus. Drizzle with the olive oil and sprinkle with the oregano. Bake for 3 minutes. Use a spatula to flip the asparagus over and bake for another 3 minutes. Serve immediately.

Rosemary Carrots   (Serves 3)

8 ounces baby carrots or large carrots cut into ½-inch pieces

extra-virgin olive oil

2 teaspoons fresh or dried rosemary leaves

Clean and peel the carrots and place them in a microwave-safe bowl. Drizzle the olive oil over the carrots and then sprinkle the rosemary leaves over them. Microwave at medium-high power for 4 minutes. The carrots will cook for another 1 or 2 minutes after being heated.

Mashed Sweet Potatoes   (Serves 4–5)

3 medium sweet potatoes (or yams)

4 tablespoons unsalted butter

4 tablespoons orange juice

¼ teaspoon salt

¼ teaspoon finely grated nutmeg

Preheat the oven to 400 degrees. Prick the sweet potatoes with a fork, place them on a baking sheet, and bake for 60 to 70 minutes. When they are cooked (somewhat soft), remove the sweet potatoes from the oven; after they have cooled a little, remove the skins with a knife. Transfer the sweet potatoes to a bowl and mash them with the other ingredients.

Wild Rice   (Serves 6)

1 cup wild rice
1 cup high-quality chicken or
   vegetable broth
2 cups water

2 stalks celery, diced
4 ounces water chestnuts, diced
2–3 tablespoons organic raisins

Rinse the rice in a strainer and transfer it to a 2-quart saucepan. Add the broth and the water. Bring to a boil over high heat (about 5 minutes) and then reduce the heat to a simmer. After 20 minutes add the celery, water chestnuts, and raisins to the rice and stir. The rice should cook fully in about 40 to 50 minutes. Fluff with a fork and drain off any excess water. The rice should be al dente; do not overcook it.

Lunch Meals

Chicken Burgers with Romano Cheese and Olives/or Shiitake Mushrooms   (Serves 4)

1 pound ground chicken
¾ cup shredded Romano cheese
6 shiitake mushrooms, diced

salt and pepper to taste
2 tablespoons extra-virgin olive oil

Thoroughly mix all the ingredients and then form patties about ½ inch thick. Heat the olive oil in a large skillet and fry the burgers on medium heat, about 3 to 4 minutes per side. The chicken burgers will be done when they feel firm when pressed with a spatula. Pat them with paper towels to blot off the extra fat. As a variation substitute 6 diced Kalamata olives in place of the mushrooms.

Simple Turkey Burgers   (Serves 4)

1 pound ground turkey
¼ cup diced red bell pepper
⅓ cup diced red or sweet yellow
   onion

4 large garlic cloves, finely diced
1 teaspoon dried oregano
1 teaspoon dried basil
salt and pepper to taste

Thoroughly mix all the ingredients and form patties about ½ inch thick. Arrange the patties on a broiling rack or tray and broil for about 5 minutes on each side, being careful not to overcook them. (Alternatively, you can pan-fry the turkey burgers in a little olive oil.) When juices run clear, the burgers will be cooked. Pat them with paper towels to blot off the extra fat. As a variation add 2 tablespoons of pine nuts or ⅓ cup of shredded Romano cheese while mixing all the ingredients together.

Chicken and Egg Salad   (Serves 4)

2 cups cooked and diced chicken (approximately ½ pound)
2 eggs, hard-boiled and diced
4 ounces water chestnuts, diced
1 tablespoon pine nuts

2 tablespoons diced sweet onion
3 tablespoons canola mayonnaise, such as Spectrum Naturals brand
2 teaspoons Dijon mustard
fresh apple wedges

Mix all the ingredients except the mayonnaise, mustard, and apple wedges. Add and stir just enough of the mayonnaise and the mustard to create a creamy texture. Serve on a bed of lettuce or baby spinach leaves, with apple wedges as a garnish.

Note: You can create a creamier texture by shredding the chicken in a food processor.

Tuna Salad   (Serves 4)

1 6-ounce can tuna (packed in water)
1 tablespoon dry-roasted unsalted cashew pieces
2 tablespoons canola mayonnaise

2 teaspoons coarse-ground French mustard
salt and freshly ground pepper to taste

Drain the tuna and place it in a bowl. With a fork, break it up into small pieces. Add the cashew pieces, mayonnaise, and mustard and mix well. Add salt and pepper.

Deli Turkey and Cheese Wrap   (Serves 1)

canola mayonnaise
1 low-carb whole-wheat tortilla
1–2 slices low-fat Jarlsberg cheese

2–3 slices deli turkey, such as Boar's Head brand

With a knife spread a little canola mayonnaise on the whole-wheat tortilla. Place the cheese and turkey on the tortilla and roll it up. Eat the wrap cold or heat it in a microwave oven for 30 to 60 seconds.

Breakfast Meals

Most of us have been acculturated to think in terms of eggs or sausage as proteins for breakfast. However, chicken and turkey, particularly leftovers from the previous night's dinner, can be added to omelettes or eaten by themselves. Enjoy these breakfasts with a side of nonstarchy fruits, such as berries or melon.

Simple, Fast Mini-Omelette   (Serves 1)

1 teaspoon extra-virgin olive oil
1 egg, beaten

1–2 tablespoons shredded (not grated) Romano, Asagio, or Mexican-style cheese

Heat the olive oil in a small nonstick skillet. Pour in the beaten egg, allowing it to form a small circle (about 4 inches in diameter). When the egg sets, in 1 to 2 minutes, use a spatula to flip it over. Sprinkle on the grated cheese and then fold the egg over. If you like, sprinkle on a small amount of a dried herb such as basil, oregano, dill, or parsley before flipping over the egg. Be careful, because the egg cooks very quickly.

Cashew and Veggie Omelette   (Serves 1)

1 teaspoon extra-virgin olive oil
1 pat of butter
1 scallion, diced
¼ red bell pepper, diced
1 tablespoon dry-roasted unsalted cashew pieces

½ cup (loosely packed) baby spinach leaves
1 tablespoon cream cheese (organic preferred)
2 eggs, beaten

In a 10-inch skillet heat the olive oil and butter over medium heat and then add the scallion, red bell pepper, and cashew pieces and sauté. When the scallion and pepper are soft, add the spinach and cream cheese and stir-fry until the spinach wilts and the cream cheese starts to melt. Transfer the sautéed vegetables temporarily to a small plate. Pour the beaten eggs into the skillet and allow them to cook until set, 1 to 2 minutes. Flip the omelette and then place the sautéed vegetables on one half and fold the omelette over them. Quantities can be doubled for two people.

Avocado and Chicken Omelette   (Serves 1)

1 teaspoon extra-virgin olive oil
1 pat of butter
2 eggs, beaten

2 tablespoons cooked and diced
  chicken pieces
½ small avocado, mashed

In a 10-inch skillet, heat the olive oil and butter over medium heat. Pour in the beaten eggs and allow them to cook until set, about 2 minutes. Flip the omelette and then place the chicken and avocado on one half and fold the omelette over. Quantities can be doubled for two people.

Breakfast Egg and Veggie Stir-Fry   (Serves 1 for 3 breakfasts)

1 tablespoon extra-virgin olive oil or
  1 very small pat of butter
3 scallions, diced
½ red bell pepper, diced
3 shiitake mushrooms (or other
  variety), diced
4 tablespoons diced leftover chicken
  or turkey, or deli turkey
1–2 artichoke hearts, diced

6 tablespoons cooked brown rice
Spice Hunter Deliciously Dill spice
  mix, to taste*
4–5 ounces fresh spinach, stems
  removed (bagged spinach is ideal)
6 eggs, beaten
2–3 tablespoons shredded Romano
  cheese

Many people don't have the time to prepare a protein-rich breakfast before work. You can make this breakfast on a Sunday morning, eat a third of it that morning, then place the other two servings in ramekins (or small bowls), cover, and refrigerate. Microwave them for breakfast on Monday and Tuesday morning.

Over medium heat, warm the olive oil in a nonstick wok and sauté the scallions, pepper, and mushrooms until they soften. Then add the turkey (or other meat), artichoke hearts, and brown rice, as well as Deliciously Dill spice mix. Stir-fry the mixture, moving it around with a spatula. Place the spinach leaves on top and allow them to soften a little before stirring the ingredients together. Add the beaten eggs and continue to stir-fry. When the eggs are just about cooked (not runny), sprinkle on the Romano cheese and let it melt. Divide the dish into three portions, placing one on your breakfast plate and two into ramekins or other small bowls to save for later. Serve with your choice of nonstarchy fresh fruit (for example, berries, kiwifruit, cantaloupe) on the side.

To vary the dish, try these substitutions: precooked baby shrimp or precooked diced pork instead of turkey; hearts of palm instead of artichoke hearts; Terrapin Ridge Wasabi Squeeze Garnishing Sauce instead of Deliciously Dill Spice Mix.

*Available at most natural food stores

Desserts

Exotic Rice Pudding   (Serves 4)

2 cups filtered or distilled water

1 cup black or purple rice
(e.g., Forbidden Rice brand†)

1 cup premium (not light) coconut
milk

3–4 teaspoons vanilla extract, or to
taste

2–3 tablespoons honey, or to taste

fresh fruit, such as banana slices or
raspberries, and whipped cream
for garnish

Bring the water to a boil over high heat in a 2-quart saucepan. Add the rice, cover, reduce the heat, and simmer for 25 to 30 minutes, until most of the water is gone. While the rice is cooking, pour the coconut milk into a mixing bowl and add 2 to 3 teaspoons of the vanilla extract and 1 to 3 tablespoons of the honey. Whisk until the honey dissolves. When the rice is done cooking and has cooled, transfer 3 cups of it to a bowl. (Save the extra rice for use as a side dish with dinner or lunch.) Add the coconut milk mixture to the rice and stir gently with a spoon. Add a little more vanilla and honey to taste. Chill the rice pudding to allow the rice time to absorb the coconut milk. Serve it topped with fruit and/or a small amount of real whipped cream.

†Lotus Foods' Forbidden Rice has a unique, rich flavor. It is available from health food or specialty food stores, or go to www.lotusfoods.com.

Greek Yogurt with Honey   (Serves 2)

8 ounces Greek yogurt‡

1–2 tablespoons honey

Divide the yogurt into two serving bowls. Drizzle on the honey and serve.

‡Available at Trader Joe's or other specialty food stores

Fresh Banana and Nut Butter   (Serves 2)

1 ripe banana   almond or peanut butter

Slice the banana into circles, each about ½ inch thick. Spread some of the nut butter onto each slice and serve.

Sample Two-Week Meal Plan

This meal plan is intended more as an idea generator rather than as a rigid diet plan for you to follow for two weeks. Most people do not have the time to cook three meals daily and instead are likely to make extensive use of leftovers. Whatever you choose to eat, however, it is important that you follow the dietary guidelines discussed in chapter 7. An asterisk (*) indicates that the recipe is included in this chapter.

Sunday   (Day 1)

Breakfast   Breakfast Egg and Veggie Stir-Fry*, fresh fruit, and black tea
Lunch   Chicken Caesar salad without croutons
Dinner   Chipotle Shrimp Fajitas*, small side salad, and sparkling water

Monday   (Day 2)

Breakfast   Breakfast Egg and Veggie Stir-Fry* (reheated), fresh fruit, and herbal tea
Lunch   Deli Turkey and Cheese Wrap*
Dinner   Salmon fillet pan-fried in olive oil, with green beans amandine

Tuesday   (Day 3)

Breakfast   Breakfast Egg and Veggie Stir-Fry* (reheated) and fresh fruit
Lunch   Tuna Salad* on a bed of lettuce
Dinner   Roasted Chicken with Rosemary and Garlic*, Sautéed Fennel, Olives, and Raisins*, and steamed green beans

Wednesday   (Day 4)

Breakfast   Avocado and Chicken Omelette* and fresh fruit
Lunch   Chef's salad without croutons
Dinner   Fillet of Sole with Almonds and Parsley*, sautéed spinach and pine nuts, and a small baked yam

Thursday   (Day 5)

Breakfast	Scrambled egg and chicken wrap in a low-carb whole-wheat tortilla
Lunch	Chicken and Egg Salad* on a bed of butter lettuce
Dinner	Shrimp with Artichoke Hearts and Dijon Sauce*, Simple Baked Asparagus*, and purple or brown rice

Friday   (Day 6)

Breakfast	Simple, Fast Mini-Omelette* and fresh fruit
Lunch	Simple Turkey Burger* (minus the bun) and side salad
Dinner	Simple Trout Amandine*, Mashed Sweet Potatoes*, and steamed broccoli and cauliflower

Saturday   (Day 7)

Breakfast	Eggs Florentine and fresh fruit
Lunch	Chicken kebab with salad
Dinner	Scallops with Saffron Sauce*, Roasted Carrots and Shallots*, and purple rice

Sunday   (Day 8)

Breakfast	Quiche Lorraine (minus the crust) and fresh fruit
Lunch	Chicken breast (minus the bun) and steamed broccoli
Dinner	Oriental-style stir-fry with finely sliced pork and vegetables

Monday   (Day 9)

Breakfast	Spinach and cheese mini-omelette
Lunch	Cobb salad
Dinner	Pan-fried salmon in olive oil and green beans almandine

Tuesday   (Day 10)

Breakfast	Slices of turkey, ham, and cheese with a fruit salad
Lunch	Beef kebab grilled with onions, cherry tomatoes, and bell peppers
Dinner	Baked turkey breast, steamed broccoli, and red rice

Wednesday (Day 11)

Breakfast   Omelette with salmon pieces

Lunch   Chicken salad on a bed of lettuce or spinach

Dinner   Fillet of sole lightly breaded with rice flour, served on top of wilted spinach, and brown rice

Thursday (Day 12)

Breakfast   Scrambled eggs with Romano cheese, with fresh fruit on the side

Lunch   Greek salad with gyro meat

Dinner   Baked cornish hens, Rosemary Carrots*, and spinach sautéed with shiitake mushrooms

Friday (Day 13)

Breakfast   Denver omelette and fresh fruit

Lunch   Smoked salmon, diced onions, and capers, along with a small tossed salad

Dinner   Baked chicken, steamed cauliflower, and brown rice

Saturday (Day 14)

Breakfast   Eggs with turkey sausage and fresh fruit on the side

Lunch   Chicken, vegetable, and brown rice soup

Dinner   Oriental-style stir-fry with shrimp and bay scallops and vegetables

Navigating Restaurant Menus

Just a few years ago, waiters and waitresses were often puzzled when customers ordered burgers without buns or steamed vegetables instead of french fries. Since then various low-carbohydrate diets have moved from the fringe to the mainstream, and many restaurants now understand and are eager to accommodate their diners' dietary preferences. Still, you will have better luck ordering foods made with high-quality, nutrient-dense ingredients at some restaurants than at others.

Although some fast-food restaurants (such as McDonald's, Burger King, and Wendy's) are making more salads and low-carb offerings available, the reality is that most of their profits come from fries and soft drinks, which are among the least healthy foods. If you are trying to adhere to a nutrient-dense diet, the smells and the temptations at fast-food restaurants may be too much to resist. There are other pitfalls as well. A healthy-looking salad may still come with a dressing high in partially hydrogenated vegetable oils, soybean oil, or cottonseed oil. It is often best simply to avoid these restaurants.

From a nutritional standpoint, national low-end chain restaurants (such as Denny's or Carrow's) are not much better than fast-food places. Nearly all the food served is manufactured before being delivered to the restaurants, and many contain various sugars, refined carbohydrates, and unhealthy oils. Again, it may be best to bypass these establishments.

You will have better luck at many ethnic restaurants, particularly Greek, Middle Eastern, Japanese, and some Italian places. Seafood and upscale new American cuisine restaurants usually offer healthy meals as well. But you must be a responsible consumer and ask questions before ordering.

They key is to avoid starchy foods (such as pastas or potatoes), deep-fried foods (such as french fries or falafel), or large amounts of white rice. Greek, Middle Eastern, and Italian restaurants typically use olive oil to cook with, and you will do best ordering chicken, fish, meats, and vegetables. If you are trying to lose weight, skip the breadbasket (simply ask the waiter to take it away). In Japanese restaurants a bowl of miso soup or a plate of sashimi (sliced raw fish) is an excellent choice; the sashimi avoids the rice that typically comes with sushi. The new American cuisine tends to be very inventive and typically uses high-quality ingredients in preparing fish, chicken, and other dishes, though such restaurants can sometimes be expensive. A baked or rotisseried half-chicken is usually a tasty and moderately priced meal.

PART IV

Nutrition Plans for Protecting and Enhancing Your Genes

9

Stress, Genes, and Nutrition

Scientists have long debated whether people are products of nature or nurture. But one does not have to be a scientist to recognize the obvious: your thoughts and emotions are shaped by *both* your initial genetic hardwiring and the many subsequent events (dietary, social, and environmental) that rewire your genes. Conversely, your emotions and thoughts directly and indirectly influence the activity of your genes, affecting your risk of disease and overall life expectancy.

Today many researchers are exploring what Ernest Rossi, Ph.D., the author of *The Psychobiology of Gene Expression*, has termed "psychosocial genomics." This merging of genetics and behavior looks at the details of how genes influence behavior and how behavior switches various genes on and off in the brain and other organs. Of particular relevance are the profound health consequences of chronic stress, a nearly pervasive feature of modern life. Stress triggers changes in hormone levels, which in turn modify the activities of multiple genes in cells throughout the body. The consequences of these genetic changes include the accelerated aging of brain cells, an increased susceptibility to depression and anxiety, and a greater long-term risk of stress-related physical illnesses, including heart disease.

This chapter describes some of the tantalizing research on the

141

interplay of genes and behavior, with an emphasis on the undesirable biochemical and genetic consequences of chronic stress. Because persistent stress is so harmful to health, this chapter also recommends specific nutritional supplements that reduce stress, apparently by increasing the activities of genes involved in neurotransmitter production. Like good wholesome foods, positive attitudes, feelings, and behavior patterns can help nourish healthy genes. On your own you can read about or take classes on a variety of stress-reducing and stress-managing lifestyle habits.

The Interplay of Genes and Behavior

Just a few years ago, scientists believed that people had a finite number of brain cells. They now understand that the brain is a dynamic, changing, and adapting organ. Experiences can increase or decrease the production of new brain cells, trigger gene transcription in brain cells leading to elevated neurotransmitter production, and reshape synapses (connections between brain cells) that influence how the brain processes information.

Genes That Increase the Risk of Depression

Some types of genetic polymorphisms (variations in the structure of genes) can heighten the risk of developing prolonged depression. As you recall from chapter 5, polymorphisms in the structure of the methylenetetrahydrofolate reductase (MTHFR) gene reduce utilization of folic acid, leading to inefficient methylation, elevated levels of homocysteine, and impaired DNA synthesis and repair. Remarkably, the same genetic variant that increases the risk of birth defects, heart disease, and cancer also increases a person's risk of depression.

In a study of almost 6,000 Norwegians, Dr. Ingvar Bjelland and colleagues from the University of Bergen found that middle-aged women with high homocysteine levels (a sign of low folic acid levels) were twice as likely to be depressed, compared with those who had normal homocysteine levels. Bjelland determined that most of the women consumed adequate amounts of dietary folic acid but that the genetic polymorphism reduced the cellular processing of the vitamin. Folic acid's role in methylation feeds into the production of neurotransmitters, brain-communication molecules involved in thinking and moods. When folic acid levels are low, or when the vitamin is not being efficiently utilized, neurotransmitter levels may decline. Conversely, considerable other research has shown that folic acid supplements may reduce depression as well as enhance the benefits of antidepressant medications.

A separate study, conducted by a team of researchers from the United States, England, and New Zealand, showed that polymorphisms in a different gene also increased a person's susceptibility to depression. Terrie E. Moffitt, Ph.D., a psychologist at King's College, London, and colleagues studied the serotonin-transporter gene in 847 subjects. This gene programs the construction of a key protein involved in moving serotonin to where it is needed in brain cells. Two versions of the gene exist, one that is longer and very efficient in transporting serotonin and one that is shorter and less efficient.

Moffitt found that people with the longer, efficient gene for transporting serotonin were not likely to become depressed after experiencing stressful life events, such as the loss of a job or the death of a family member. However, people with one copy (from one parent) or two copies (from both parents) of the shorter, less efficient form of the gene were far more likely to experience depression. Thirty-three percent of people with one copy of the short gene became depressed, and 43 percent of people with two copies of the short gene became depressed after experiencing stressful life events.

Moffitt's research is particularly interesting because nearly all pharmaceutical treatments for depression, including Prozac and Zoloft, are intended to enhance serotonin levels in brain cells. Similarly, many natural treatments for depression also focus on improved utilization of serotonin. For example, the amino acids tryptophan and 5-hydroxy-tryptophan (5-HTP) are the biochemical precursors to serotonin, and considerable research supports their benefits in the treatment of depression and anxiety. It is plausible that people with the short serotonin-transporter gene are more likely to benefit from tryptophan or 5-HTP supplements. These two natural substances may help "load" the genes and biochemical pathways involved in serotonin synthesis and transport, just as folic acid supplements improve the activity of a sluggish MTHFR gene.

How Shelley Solved Her Blues

Shelley, age fifty, began having serious bouts of depression and overreacting to the usual stresses of running her business. A physician prescribed an antidepressant drug, which resulted in her gaining weight but did not completely resolve her depression and anxiety. He prescribed a second antidepressant drug, but it didn't help.

When Shelley went to a nutritionally oriented physician, he tested her urine for kryptopyrrole, a chemical that binds to and excretes vitamin B_6 and zinc, two nutrients that influence mood. Shelly tested positive for this genetic predisposition, and work-related stresses increased her production of kryptopyrrole and loss of vitamin B_6 and zinc. The effect was comparable to a deficiency of both nutrients.

Her physician recommended a high-potency B-complex supplement, containing 100 mg of the major B vitamins. He also suggested that she take extra vitamin B_6 and inositol (a B vitamin helpful in depression and anxiety), as well as zinc supplements. Within two weeks Shelley's depression lifted, and she now remains calm in the face of work pressures.

She has also had a number of "side benefits," including higher energy levels, better concentration, greater self-confidence, and more restful sleep. Because of her increased energy, Shelley has started to cook more foods from scratch and is eating more fish and vegetables. She has also lost her sweet tooth, along with ten pounds in two months. "I haven't felt this good in years," she says.

Behaviors That Modify Genes and Brain Structure

Prenatal influences and early childhood development can have lasting effects on a person's long-term mental and physical health. But rather than being strictly a behavioral consequence, as psychologists have generally believed, these experiences actually affect gene activity in brain cells, the creation of new brain cells, and the hardwiring of a child's developing brain.

For example, several teams of researchers have shown that prenatal and infant stresses reduce DNA synthesis and the production of new brain cells, leading to smaller brain sizes and more fearful behavior later in life. At the University of Wisconsin, researchers exposed pregnant rhesus monkeys, close biological relatives of humans, to regular stresses, such as loud and startling sounds. The monkeys' offspring, more than two years after birth, exhibited elevated levels of cortisol, one of the body's prime stress hormones, reduced formation of brain cells in some regions of the brain, and smaller brains.

Similarly, animal studies by Michael J. Meaney, Ph.D., of McGill University in Montreal have shown that normal maternal care, such as a mother rodent's licking and grooming her pups, bolstered the pups' long-term resistance to stress and stress-induced illness. In contrast, the absence of this behavior increased the pups' stress and led to higher levels of pituitary and adrenal hormones, particularly cortisol. These stress-related hormonal changes initiated a cascade of permanent alterations in DNA structure and stress responses, eventually increasing susceptibility to stress-related diseases. Although similar controlled studies would not be ethical with human subjects, observational studies have found that a lack of regular contact between mother and child can lead to aloof, fearful, and abnormal behavior in children.

A multitude of other factors also affect brain development and the activities of genes in brain cells. For example, some researchers have proposed that the hormone insulin has effects similar to those of testosterone in gene activity and the organization of the fetal brain. Like testosterone, insulin stimulates the growth of various types of brain cells as well as synapses, and elevated insulin levels may program brain cells for increased appetite and body weight.

Alcoholic beverages, which influence behavior, also modify gene activity, according to research by R. Adron Harris, Ph.D., the director of the Waggoner Center for Alcohol and Addiction Research at the University of Texas. Harris and his colleagues analyzed the activity of ten thousand genes in two regions in the brains of alcoholics. They found that alcohol altered the activity of 191 genes, particularly those involved in judgment and decision making. Among the affected genes were those that have a role in the production of myelin, which forms a protective sheath around nerve cells. Damage to the myelin sheath, which also occurs in multiple sclerosis, can literally short-circuit the transmission of nerve and brain signals. Thus, alcohol consumption appears to do far more than just temporarily impair judgment and reflexes. It actually changes the behavior of genes in the brain.

Even negative emotions and so-called sour moods can stimulate the secretion of cortisol and adrenaline and reduce the production of serotonin. Brooding about bad things that have happened to you in life, being irritable, or harboring resentment and anger all help sustain a stress-hormone response. In the long term, such bad moods can suppress normal DNA synthesis, reduce production of new brain cells, and reshape brain-cell connections in undesirable ways, helping set the stage for chronic depression or anxiety.

One of the unhealthiest clusters of emotional traits consists of a combination of aggressiveness, mistrust, and anger—what psychologists define as a "hostile personality." People with hostile personalities tend to experience an especially strong stress response, characterized by elevated cortisol levels, and they are seven times more likely to die at a younger age. Like alcohol, the intensity of this behavior can suppress genes involved in normal thinking processes and healthy emotional expression. Increasing intake of the nutritional building blocks of neurotransmitters often can help reset brain chemistry and promote calmer behavior. (See "Nutrients That Reduce Stress" later in this chapter.)

Antidepressant Drugs Boost Gene Activity in the Brain

One of the recent surprises in psychosocial genomics has been a better understanding of how antidepressant drugs act on the brain. For years physicians thought that antidepressant drugs, such as Prozac, work primarily by improving cellular regulation of the neurotransmitter serotonin. But research increasingly points to another mode of action: that at least some antidepressant drugs actually stimulate the synthesis of new DNA, brain cells, and connections between brain cells, a process called neurogenesis.

Prozac and other antidepressant drugs, as well as the herb St. John's wort, begin boosting serotonin levels almost immediately. By doing so, they should rapidly relieve depression. However, these therapies typically take two to four weeks to have a noticeable effect, suggesting that they work by another mechanism.

This delay in exerting an antidepressant effect has led some researchers, such as Rene Hen, Ph.D., of the National Institute of Mental Health, to investigate whether these drugs might actually work by generating new brain cells and synapses between brain cells, a process that takes several weeks. Hen and several teams of researchers have shown that antidepressant drugs do in fact increase neurogenesis. In experiments Hen has shown that antidepressant medications lead to a 60 percent increase in a key chemical marker of neurogenesis.

This research indicates that changes in DNA synthesis (required for new cells) or gene activity lie behind many, if not most, of the biochemical changes that occur in the brain (and likely the body as a whole). In a very real sense, nearly everything that happens in our bodies ultimately takes place on a genetic level.

The Cascading Health Effects of Stress

The stress response is one of the oldest and most universal biological reactions to danger. It is deeply ingrained in both people and other animals, because for tens of millions of years, survival depended on quick reflexes and reactions to dangerous situations, such as being chased by predators.

Stress Response and Stress Hormones

Stressful experiences trigger the nearly instant release of adrenaline and glucocorticoid hormones, such as cortisol, from the adrenal glands. These hormones in turn almost instantly shut down genes and metabolic activities involved in most long-term physiological processes, such as digestion, growth, healing, and reproduction. At the same time, increased genetic activity immediately shifts nearly all the body's biochemical resources to the heart and skeletal muscles for either fighting or running, the well-known fight-or-flight stress response. In the wild, animals experience this type of stress only occasionally and only for brief periods—often less than a minute—such as when a deer is being chased by a cougar. The deer's body literally marshals all its resources to run for its life. If the deer successfully escapes, its adrenaline and cortisol levels quickly return to normal.

This stress response—the biological equivalent of going from zero to sixty in a second or two—was designed only for brief reactions to danger. When it is sustained for long periods, as it often is in modern society, the health consequences can be disastrous. Stress hormones affect virtually every organ in the body, leading to chronic inflammation, slow healing, high blood pressure, reduced circulation, and coronary artery disease. Stress accelerates the aging of cells, particularly brain cells, it suppresses DNA synthesis, and it interferes with thinking and memory. It sets the biochemical stage for depression, anxiety, and, in a severe form, posttraumatic stress disorder.

When the brain is chronically exposed to stress hormones, genes turn on and off in response to unfamiliar stimuli. These hormones, at high levels for long periods of time, can even be neurotoxic, leading to an inhibition of neurogenesis and to brain damage and brain shrinkage. As but one example, cortisol interferes with the activity of "brain-derived neurotrophic factor," a chemical that promotes neurogenesis. Memory problems can be one consequence of these undesirable changes in the brain.

Stress and Inflammation

Chronic stress can also set the stage for inflammatory diseases, contributing to arthritis, obesity, diabetes, heart disease, and many other diseases. By activating the sympathetic nervous system, stress triggers a cascade of hormonal and chemical changes that promote chronic inflammation. Some of the hormonal changes lead to the increased production of cytokines, cell-communication molecules that include interleukin-6 and C-reactive protein. These cytokines signal immune cells to release other inflammation-promoting compounds, such as prostaglandin E2—one of the body's most potent promoters of inflammation. Underlying all of these biochemical changes are fundamental alterations in gene activity, because genes ultimately program the production of these biochemicals.

As I explained in *The Inflammation Syndrome*, chronic inflammation is involved in virtually every degenerative disease, including obesity, diabetes, and heart disease. Cortisol and other stress hormones increase the deposition of fat, particularly around the belly. Abdominal fat cells exacerbate the situation because they secrete large amounts of interleukin-6 and C-reactive protein, which help maintain both low-grade inflammation and the body's stress response.

Protecting Yourself from Stress-Related Brain Damage

Scientists have gained an excellent understanding of the health consequences of chronic stress, and over the years many alternative and complementary practitioners have recommended a variety of stress-reducing activities, such as deep breathing, yoga, and meditation. Recently, in *The Psychobiology of Gene Expression: Neuroscience and Neurogenesis in Hypnosis and the Healing Arts*, Ernest Rossi, Ph.D., developed a conceptual framework for activities that not only reduce stress but also promote the growth of new and healthy brain cells and synapses between neurons. The underlying idea is this: if stress can lead to deleterious changes in brain cells, such as the inhibition of neurogenesis, positive and life-enriching activities should foster the growth of new brain cells and new connections between brain cells.

It turns out that creative endeavors and other positive life experiences can promote neurogenesis. Writing in a medical journal, Rossi explained that three general types of activities have been shown to promote normal gene expression, neurogenesis, and healing. These experiences involve novelty, environmental enrichment, and exercise. Novelty includes exposure to new and satisfying experiences, such as travel in another country. Environmental enrichment includes creative pursuits, such as learning how to draw or attending a musical concert.

Exercise is known to increase production of muscle cells and energy levels, but it also boosts levels of neurotransmitters such as serotonin. Amazingly, changes in gene activity and brain cells begin taking place within ten minutes of starting an activity and can continue for hours.

There is a good chance you believe that the stresses in your life are inevitable or unavoidable. However, it is usually possible to moderate your reaction to specific stresses and to relax. When you reduce the stress—or your response to it—you lessen stress-induced hormonal changes and subsequent damage to brain cells. But there is a catch: you must be willing to make some changes in your habits and attitudes.

Nutrients That Reduce Stress

As you have already read, many nutrients are involved in the synthesis and repair of DNA, processes essential for the manufacture of new cells, including brain cells. Many of these same nutrients also serve as the chemical building blocks of neurotransmitters or coenzymes involved in neurotransmitter production.

Chronic stress places a greater demand on these nutrients and can diminish their levels. One consequence is an inhibition of both DNA synthesis and the production of new brain cells. Stress can also reduce neurotransmitter production and set the stage for depression, anxiety, or panic attacks. When chronic stress is combined with nutrient deficiencies because of poor eating habits, the risk of mood disorders can increase sharply.

A healthy diet and certain nutritional supplements create a friendly environment for normal neurotransmitter production, as well as the production of new DNA and cells, in the brain. Nutritious foods and supplements strengthen the biochemical underpinnings of the brain.

Eating Habits. When you eat too many sugars and refined carbohydrates, or when you skip a meal, you can feel your blood sugar drop. Low blood sugar impairs your concentration and judgment, leaves you tired and fuzzy-headed, and sometimes makes you feel irritable. These symptoms often vanish after you eat something and your blood sugar rises.

Unfortunately, the typical American diet is rich in sugary foods and refined carbohydrates, which are rapidly digested and quickly boost blood-sugar levels. But this sudden elevation in blood sugar triggers the rapid secretion of insulin, a hormone that lowers blood-sugar levels. The result is a roller-coaster effect, with the ups and downs (and low-blood-sugar symptoms) occurring within a couple of hours. In addition, high-carbohydrate foods lower the levels of vitamin B_1, which is needed to break down carbohydrates for energy.

Large amounts of coffee and other caffeine-containing beverages (such as colas) compound the problem, in large part because they also contain various sugars. Even without sugar, caffeine-containing beverages trigger the release of stored sugar (glycogen) from the liver, with the effect being similar to that of having a soft drink and a doughnut. Is it any wonder that people's impatience and irritability have appeared to increase along with the number of Starbucks and drive-through cafés?

One part of the solution is emphasizing a diet rich in protein and nonstarchy, high-fiber vegetables, as described in chapter 7. Both protein and fiber help stabilize blood-sugar and insulin levels, which will then help even out mood swings. The protein provides at least two benefits: it has little effect on blood-sugar levels, and some of the amino acids derived from it are used to construct neurotransmitters. Fiber slows the absorption of carbohydrates, thus moderating the swings in blood-sugar and insulin levels.

B Vitamins. Discussed in chapter 5, the B-complex family of vitamins has long been known as the antistress nutrients. Some of the B vitamins are involved in DNA-synthesis and -repair processes, necessary for the production of new cells in the brain and throughout the body. Many of the B vitamins, such as vitamin B_6, are needed for the body's production of brain-calming neurotransmitters, such as serotonin, taurine, and gamma-amino butyric acid (GABA).

David Benton, Ph.D., a professor at the University of Wales, found that 50 mg of vitamin B_1 daily helped otherwise healthy young adults feel more "composed and energetic." In a separate study, Benton found that a daily high-potency multivitamin helped improve the moods of young women. The benefits seemed most related to vitamins B_2 and B_6 in the multivitamin supplement.

Similarly, prison studies conducted by Stephen J. Schoenthaler, Ph.D., a sociology professor at California State University, have found that a simple multivitamin supplement, or replacing candy with fruit, reduces the incidence of violence among incarcerated teenagers and adults. Schoenthaler believes that proper nutrition improves the connections between brain cells.

If you tend to be depressed or edgy, take a high-potency B-complex supplement that includes 25 to 50 mg of vitamin B_1.

Inositol. When we're stressed, it's easy to become panicky and overreact to situations. Several clinical studies have found that inositol, a nutrient related to B vitamins, can be of great benefit in panic attacks, depression, and obsessive-compulsive disorder. In a study at Israel's Barzilai Medical Center, Dr. Jonathan Benjamin compared inositol to an antidepressant drug in 21 patients who had frequent panic attacks. After one month of taking 12 to 18 grams of inositol daily, patients had significantly fewer panic attacks. They also had fewer side effects compared with people taking the drug.

To achieve Benjamin's 12 to 18 grams of inositol daily, you would have to take at least that many tablets or capsules. Your best source for such a product would be a compounding pharmacy, a drugstore that makes custom preparations. However, you may gain comparable benefits by taking 2 to 5 grams of inositol daily in combination with a high-potency B-complex supplement, available at any health food store.

Vitamin C. When your intake of vitamin C is low, a situation that affects as much as 30 percent of Americans, you are more apt to feel fatigued and irritable. Brain cells are rich in vitamin C, which help temper stress reactions by modulating catecholamines (brain chemicals) and other neurotransmitters. In a recent study, Dr. Stuart Brody of the University of Trier in Germany found that vitamin C supplements (3,000 mg daily) improved the overall mood of patients and led to more frequent and satisfying sexual activity.

Vitamin C is crucial to health, and most people do not consume enough of it. Take a minimum of 500 mg of supplemental vitamin C daily. A more ideal dosage, divided up once or twice during the day, would be 1,000 to 3,000 mg. Read the fine print on the label carefully to avoid products with added sugars (including lactose).

Theanine. Although found in green tea, which contains caffeine, theanine has a powerful anticaffeine, brain-calming effect. In fact, theanine (an amino acid) may account for the many health benefits of tea, from promoting relaxation to lowering the risk of heart disease and cancer. Some research suggests that theanine might also lower blood pressure, one consequence of stress.

Theanine supplements are available in health foods stores. Follow label directions, because products vary. Another and more preferable option is to simply drink one or two cups of green tea daily.

Gamma-Amino Butyric Acid (GABA). This amino acid also functions as a neurotransmitter, and nutritionally oriented physicians often use GABA to treat anxiety. A study by researchers at the University of

Utah School of Medicine identified part of the mechanism. GABA helps the brain filter out distracting signals—background noise, so to speak—that impair thinking. For use as a supplement, take 500 to 4,000 mg of GABA daily.

Tryptophan and 5-Hydroxy-Tryptophan (5-HTP). During the 1980s tryptophan, an essential amino acid, became a popular natural tranquilizer, sleep aid, and remedy for depression. Then, after hundreds of people were sickened by a single contaminated batch of tryptophan (imported from Japan) in 1989, the Food and Drug Administration overreacted and banned it as an over-the-counter supplement.

Today tryptophan supplements are available only by prescription in the United States. Ironically, it is necessary for health, remarkably safe, and legally must still be added to baby formulas. Nonprescription tryptophan supplements have been replaced by 5-HTP, a closely related compound that is a precursor to serotonin. Like tryptophan, 5-HTP has brain-calming, antianxiety, and antidepressant benefits—and an exceptional record of safety. For use as a supplement, take 300 to 400 mg before bedtime.

In the next chapter, we will consider the genetic components of some common physical diseases and behavioral disorders, as well as the specific nutrients that enhance gene function in these conditions.

10

Nutritional Recommendations for Specific Diseases, A to Z

Up to this point, we have focused on describing what is largely a generic, or widely applicable, nutrition and lifestyle plan for maintaining optimal gene function. In this chapter we focus more specifically on the relationship between genes and individual diseases and conditions. These diseases and conditions involve (1) inborn genetic mutations or variations, (2) acquired genetic damage, or (3) a combination of both factors.

From a practical standpoint, the difficulty often becomes defining (and diagnosing) what is and is not a disease. For example, osteoporosis and cancer are obviously diseases. But is an inherited polymorphism in the vitamin D receptor (VDR) that may increase the risk of osteoporosis or cancer a disease as well? The question is not an easy one to answer. We all are born with genetic variations or acquire genetic damage that increases our risk of disease. A VDR-gene polymorphism may help identify risk, but it cannot foretell disease with absolute certainty. The risk associated with a VDR-gene polymorphism can be easily offset by spending more time in the sun (prompting the body's manufacture of vitamin D) or by taking vitamin D supplements.

The definition of what is and is not a disease is in transition, a situation that begs us to be cautious in equating a genetic predisposition with an actual disease. In an article in the journal *Science*, Dr. James G. Wright, a professor of surgery at Toronto's Hospital for Sick Children, wrote that "disease is a fluid concept influenced by societal and cultural attitudes that change with time and in response to new scientific and medical discoveries." A case in point: in many societies people who experience visions and hallucinations have been considered prophets or shamans, but in Western nations such people are often diagnosed as schizophrenic.

In trying to redefine the meaning of disease, Wright suggested that a disease should consist of three elements: "*a state* that places individuals at *increased risk* of *adverse consequences*." This approach tempers the desire to classify all genetic variations as diseases, particularly when the risk of such diseases can be modified through dietary and lifestyle changes. Instead it considers whether the genetic variations pose a *risk* of disease.

We begin by discussing the aging process, which reflects accumulated damage to genes and other cell structures. Whether aging is or is not an actual disease remains arguable. However, aging does entail widespread genetic damage, which increases the risk of chronic degenerative diseases, including Alzheimer's disease, cardiovascular diseases, and cancer.

Aging

What Happens

Aging is the most common genetic disorder, and it affects every living creature. It reflects the overall deterioration of our DNA, genes, nongenetic cell structures, and biochemical processes. Until about age twenty-seven for most people, their gene-repair mechanisms, along with normal growth processes, stay ahead of ongoing damage to genes. After this time gene damage begins to outpace repair mechanisms, and people begin a slow but accelerating decline toward senescence. Some tissues, such as those that form your heart, brain, or skin, may age faster than others.

Some specific genes are associated with an increased risk of age-related diseases, such as the APOE E4 gene in heart disease and the BRCA1 and BRCA2 genes in breast cancer. Conversely, some genes, such as the -1082 GG gene, are associated with increased longevity and resistance to chronic inflammation. However, no single gene appears to play a governing role in the aging process. Rather, aging reflects widespread damage to large numbers of different genes, ultimately leading to a total cessation of activity.

The Gene Connection

Although theories of aging differ, most point to accumulated damage to DNA, which impairs the normal functioning of genes. The most widely held theory of aging centers on the destructive molecules called free radicals, which primarily leak out of energy-producing chemical reactions in cells. These chemical reactions are necessary for life—they break down blood sugar and fats for energy—and so life, ironically, contains the seeds for age-related gene damage and death. Other free radicals form as a result of detoxification activities, such as breaking down air pollutants and pesticides, as well as of immune activity, such as when white blood cells use free radicals to destroy infectious bacteria.

As people age and acquire genetic damage, their genes become less stable and reliable, leading to incorrect genetic programming and increased cellular malfunctioning. The two most common causes of death in developed nations are heart disease and cancer, both of which reflect gene-based defects in immune function and related biochemistry. Neither heart disease nor cancer—or any other age-related degenerative disease, for that matter—results from the failure of a single gene. Rather, age-related diseases develop from what could best be described as a genetic "system failure" involving damage to dozens, and often hundreds, of different genes.

The first target of free radicals is the nearest: mitochondrial DNA, which largely programs energy production. As mitochondrial genes are damaged, energy production becomes less efficient, leading to the creation of still more free radicals. These free radicals react with and damage proteins and fats in the cell, as well as with nuclear DNA, the source of most of our genes.

At the same time, a multiplicity of other deleterious changes occur. Consumption of excess calories, particularly starches and sugars, increases both blood-glucose and insulin levels. Glucose, particularly when elevated to prediabetic and diabetic levels, autooxidizes—that is, begins a chain reaction that generates more free radicals. Meanwhile, elevated levels of insulin promote the activity of a variety of genes involved in inflammation and stress-hormone responses. This gene activity may be increased further through injuries and infections and by psychological stresses.

Inflammation, while necessary to protect against infection and to initiate healing, may become systemic, particularly if the diet is low in antioxidants and antiinflammatory fats (such as omega-3 fish oils and gamma-linolenic acid). In fact, low-grade inflammation is known to increase with age, partly reflecting increased immune-cell activity to dispose of aging, malfunctioning, and dead cells. Chronic psychological stresses increase levels of the stress hormone cortisol, which in turn elevates blood glucose and insulin and helps set the stage for abdominal obesity.

What You Can Do

With this age-related genetic deterioration comes a decline in our assimilation and utilization of all nutrients. Because nutrients are the most basic building blocks for each of the body's other biochemicals, the consequences of this growing inefficiency cascade can affect every aspect of health. For example, levels of most hormones decline with age, bone density cannot be maintained and decreases, the number of muscle cells decreases, and the immune system's ability to resist infection decreases.

Two steps can significantly slow the age-related accumulation of free-radical damage. One is building up and maintaining, over many years, a nutritional reserve that improves your body's ability to resist genetic and nongenetic cell damage. The other way is to "load" cells with specific nutrients, such as B vitamins and free-radical-neutralizing antioxidants, to enhance DNA functioning and to reduce damage.

The nutritional-reserve concept is a long-term strategy for minimizing DNA and cell damage. It is best applied as early as possible in life, though it can provide striking benefits at any age. The dietary guidelines in chapter 7 describe a nutrient-dense diet, emphasizing quality protein and fresh nonstarchy vegetables, which supports this nutritional reserve. Many studies have shown that variations of this diet, such as the Mediterranean diet, reduce the risk of heart disease and cancer. Following this type of diet can also help you look younger as well as feel younger. In one recent study, researchers have reported that people who ate diets rich in fish, vegetables, and olive oil had fewer skin wrinkles compared with people who consumed sugary soft drinks, pastries, and potatoes.

Many studies have shown that nutritional supplements can effectively load the body's cells and reduce DNA, gene, and chromosome damage. Nutrient loading is comparable to saturating gene-dependent biochemical pathways in the body. This approach does work—human studies routinely find that blood and tissue levels of nutrients increase after supplementation, usually with improvements in clinical symptoms. Genetic polymorphisms that increase the risk of disease are also responsive to higher levels of nutrients. For example, supplemental folic acid and vitamin D offset polymorphisms that reduce the metabolism of these vitamins. By loading or saturating the genes' biochemical pathways, inefficient genes are given the ability to function normally and prevent disease. The effect of *not* maintaining high levels of vitamins and minerals, through either diet or supplements, has the same net cellular effect as radiation damage to DNA, according to the eminent cell biologist Bruce N. Ames, Ph.D., of the University of California at Berkeley. That alone is a compelling reason to supplement. And although many nutrients (except refined starches and sugars) are essential for health, those discussed in chapters 4, 5, and 6 are especially important.

It is difficult to design or recommend a single supplement that will suit every lifestyle or health concern. For the sake of relative simplicity, the following dietary supplement provides moderately high levels of the nutrients needed to ensure normal functioning of your genes and cells.

—⁂—

An "Ideal" Daily Supplement

If you want to maintain (or improve) your health with relatively few pills and capsules, shop for a supplement that contains all or most of the following vitamins and minerals, and strive for the dosage recommendations. Although this formula does not represent a real product, you should be able to find comparable multivitamin and multimineral supplements. When shopping, ask for a high-potency multivitamin supplement and a regular-potency mineral supplement. The vitamin-like nutrients will likely have to be purchased as individual supplements.

VITAMINS

vitamin A	5,000 IU
vitamin B_1	10–50 mg
vitamin B_2	10–50 mg
vitamin B_3	10–75 mg
vitamin B_6	10–75 mg
vitamin B_{12}	75–500 mcg
biotin	75–200 mcg

choline	50–100 mg
folic acid	400–800 mcg
inositol	50–100 mg
pantothenic acid	75–100 mg
vitamin C*	500–3,000 mg
vitamin D	400–800 IU
vitamin E	200–400 IU
vitamin K	50–100 mcg

MINERALS

calcium*	800–1,000 mg
chromium*	200–400 mcg
copper	2–4 mg
iodine	50–150 mcg
iron[†]	0–10 mg
manganese	5–10 mg
magnesium	200–400 mg
phosphorus[‡]	0 mg
potassium	10–50 mg
selenium	200 mcg
zinc	15–30 mg

VITAMIN-LIKE NUTRIENTS

coenzyme Q10*	30–100 mg
carnitine*	500–1,000 mg
alpha-lipoic acid*	50–100 mg
carotenoids	10–20 mg
flavonoids	100–200 mg

*Individual supplements (rather than multiples) will likely be required to achieve these dosages.

[†]Men and postmenopausal women may not need supplemental iron. People with hemochromatosis or other iron-storage disorders should not take any supplemental iron.

[‡]Although phosphorus is an essential nutrient, it is not usually required supplementally, because most foods (as a result of high-phosphorus fertilizers) are typically rich in this mineral.

Alzheimer's Disease

What Happens

Alzheimer's disease is the most common type of dementia (senility) and accounts for about two-thirds of all cases. An estimated 4 million Americans currently have some degree of Alzheimer's disease. The Chicago-based Alzheimer's Foundation predicts that more than 14 million people will have the disease by the year 2050. While these numbers may be inflated, the prevalence of Alzheimer's disease is likely to grow as the overall population ages.

Symptomatically, Alzheimer's disease is characterized by a severe deterioration in memory combined with a decline in at least one other cognitive function, such as language skills, perceptions, or emotional reactions. In later stages it leads to a loss of motor skills and independence in day-to-day activities, such as grooming and going to the bathroom. Because an accurate diagnosis can be determined only by autopsy, physicians use a variety of criteria to assess whether a senile patient has "probable" Alzheimer's disease.

On a biochemical level, Alzheimer's disease is characterized by clumps and tangles of beta-amyloid protein around brain cells. Beta-amyloid protein interferes with normal brain-cell activity as well as with the production of new brain cells.

Cerebrovascular disease is the second most common cause of dementia. Ministrokes reduce blood flow to various regions of the brain and increase localized production of harmful free radicals. Brain injury from cerebrovascular disease sometimes overlaps with the beta-amyloid deposits characteristic of Alzheimer's disease.

The Gene Connection

Researchers have identified several genes that are strongly associated with early-onset Alzheimer's disease, which is relatively rare. These genes are not usually present in the more common late-onset Alzheimer's disease.

However, the apolipoprotein E4 (APOE E4) gene has been consistently associated with a higher risk of late-onset Alzheimer's disease. Apolipoprotein E is a constituent of low-density lipoprotein (LDL), the blood's carrier of vitamin E, vitamin A, and carotenoids. People with the APOE E4 gene also have elevated cholesterol levels and a higher risk of coronary heart disease. However, not every person with this gene will develop Alzheimer's disease, suggesting that other genes, dietary factors, and lifestyle habits influence the risk of Alzheimer's disease.

Elevated levels of homocysteine are strongly associated with an increased risk of Alzheimer's disease. In fact, people with blood levels of homocysteine above 14 micromoles per liter of blood are two to four times more likely to develop Alzheimer's disease, compared with those who have normal homocysteine levels. In general, the elevated homocysteine is related more to low intake of folic acid and other B vitamins rather than to variations in the gene coding for methylenetetrahydrofolate reductase. Abnormally high levels of homocysteine, a consequence of low B-vitamin intake, is toxic to brain cells and also damages blood vessels in the brain.

Growing evidence points to chronic low-grade cerebral inflammation as a cause of Alzheimer's disease. Such inflammation may be the result of serious brain injuries earlier in life. During the inflammatory reaction to injury, the body produces large numbers of free radicals, which stimulate the formation of beta-amyloid protein in the brain.

What You Can Do

Vitamin E

Several studies have found that high intake of vitamin E, in either foods or supplements, can reduce the risk of developing Alzheimer's disease. The vitamin helps neutralize free radicals, has mild antiinflammatory properties, and also protects brain cells from beta-amyloid protein.

Martha Clare Morris, Sc.D., of the Rush–Presbyterian–St. Luke's Medical Center in Chicago found that high intake of vitamin E reduced the risk of Alzheimer's disease by 70 percent. However, people with the APOE E4 gene, which increases the risk of Alzheimer's disease, were most likely to benefit from the vitamin. A more recent study by Peter P. Zandi, Ph.D., of Johns Hopkins University found similar benefits among people who had taken vitamin E and C supplements.

In a Dutch study of 5,395 people, Dr. Marianne J. Engelhart of the Erasmus Medical Center in Rotterdam reported that high dietary intake of vitamin E reduced the risk of Alzheimer's disease by 18 percent overall. However, smokers who ate a lot of vitamin E–rich foods reduced their risk of Alzheimer's disease by 42 percent.

Very large dosages of vitamin E (2,000 IU daily) have also been shown to slow the progression of late-stage Alzheimer's disease, according to a large clinical trial by Mary Sano, Ph.D., of the Columbia

University College of Physicians and Surgeons. Although the subjects' cognitive functions did not improve, they were able to take care of themselves (such as performing personal grooming) much longer compared with patients taking a placebo. In a follow-up study, Sano is trying to determine whether vitamin E supplements will slow the progression of Alzheimer's disease in its early stages.

ALPHA-LIPOIC ACID

A serendipitous discovery by German physicians found that daily supplements of alpha-lipoic acid (600 mg) might halt cognitive decline in Alzheimer's disease. The physicians used alpha-lipoic acid to treat diabetic complications in a patient also diagnosed with mild Alzheimer's disease. The patient's cognitive functions stabilized after regular alpha-lipoic acid supplementation. Dr. Klaus Hager and his colleagues used alpha-lipoic acid to treat eight other mild-to-moderate Alzheimer's disease patients for one year. Using standard medical tests for assessing the disease, Hager found that the patients' cognitive functions remained stable during this time. Normally their cognitive skills would have declined appreciably.

Animal studies conducted at Oregon State University have found that a combination of alpha-lipoic acid and acetyl-L-carnitine (a form of carnitine) can improve memory and lead to a partial reversal of the aging process. These two nutrients, described in chapter 4, reduce free-radical damage to both DNA and RNA *and* increase energy activity in brain cells.

VITAMIN B_{12} AND FOLIC ACID

Both nutrients lower blood levels of homocysteine and are involved in the body's production of new DNA and cells. Low levels of either folic acid or vitamin B_{12} doubled the risk of developing Alzheimer's disease, according to research by Hui-Xin Wang, Ph.D., of the Karolinska Instutute in Stockholm. Conversely, maintaining normal to high intake of these nutrients, through diet or supplements, reduced the risk of Alzheimer's disease. In fact, some cases of dementia may be caused by nothing more than a deficiency of vitamin B_{12}, which is easily corrected through supplementation.

GINKGO BILOBA

This herbal remedy, long recommended for improving memory, has been shown to increase the activity of ten key genes in the brain, influencing memory, speech, logical thinking, and emotional responses. Its benefits in slowing Alzheimer's disease, while not always consistent, are extremely promising. In a study using a proprietary extract of ginkgo, Dr. Pierre L. LeBars of the New York Institute for Medical Research found that the herb (EGb 761 extract, 40 mg three times daily) moderately increased cognitive performance and social functioning in patients suffering from dementia.

Birth Defects

What Happens

Birth defects result from significant alterations in DNA and genes during the growth and development of a fetus. Pregnant women who consume low levels of vitamins have an increased risk of delivering a child with some types of birth defects. This section focuses on several common birth defects that can be prevented, or ameliorated after birth, through improved diet and supplements.

CLEFT LIP AND PALATE

A cleft lip, which is relatively common, is a split in the middle of the upper lip, whereas a cleft palate is characterized by a hole in the roof of the mouth. Together they are among the most common of all birth defects.

SPINA BIFIDA

In spina bifida, the neural tube, which develops into the brain and spine, fails to close during the first month of gestation. Very mild cases may be identified by only a tuft of hair at the bottom of the spine. In more severe cases, the spinal cord is exposed at birth. Nerve damage, paralysis of the lower body, and a lack of bladder control are common consequences of spina bifida. Other types of neural-tube defects include encephalocele, in which the brain protrudes through the skull, and anencephaly, the complete absence of the brain and spinal column.

DOWN SYNDROME

This common genetic disorder is characterized by the existence of a third copy of the twenty-first chromosome (and all of the genes normally found on that chromosome). It results in "mongoloid" physical features, mental retardation, a greater risk of developing leukemia and early-onset Alzheimer's disease, and reduced life expectancy. Although the underlying genetic disorder causing Down syndrome cannot be changed, many of the associated biochemical problems can be circumvented through high-dose vitamin and mineral supplements and thyroid medications, leading to improved intelligence and appearance.

CHILDHOOD BRAIN CANCER

Although technically not a birth defect, the development of brain cancer early in life points to subtle, as-yet-unidentified prenatal defects or damage to brain-cell DNA. At least nine studies have shown that pregnant women who eat large amounts of N-nitroso compounds, found in hot dogs and many luncheon meats, have children with a substantially higher risk of brain cancer.

The Gene Connection

Women who carry polymorphisms in the gene programming for methylenetetrahydrofolate reductase (MTHFR), and who do not consume adequate amounts of folic acid (and other B vitamins), are more likely to have children with cleft lip, cleft palate, and spina bifida. As you read in chapter 5, folic acid and several other B vitamins play fundamental roles in the production of DNA, needed for the creation of new cells. During pregnancy a woman's folic acid requirements increase substantially to support the rapid growth of her fetus.

CLEFT LIP AND PALATE

Regine P. M. Steegers-Theunissen, Ph.D., of University Medical Center in the Netherlands recently compared the dietary habits of the mothers of 179 women who delivered children with a cleft lip, a cleft palate, or both conditions with mothers of 204 children without the birth defects. Steegers-Theunissen reported in the *Journal of Epidemiology* that women with polymorphisms in the MTHFR gene, who also consumed low levels of dietary or supplemental folic acid, were six to seven times more likely to deliver a child with cleft lip or palate.

SPINA BIFIDA

In the 1960s researchers in Wales noted that women with low dietary intake of folic acid were more likely to have children with spina bifida and other neural-tube defects. It took until the late 1980s for medical journals and professional medical societies to officially recognize the fundamental importance of folic acid in preventing spina bifida. More recent research has shown, not surprisingly, that some MTHFR polymorphisms may increase the risk of spina bifida, most likely by reducing folic acid activity. In addition, animal studies have clearly shown that an elevated level of homocysteine (the result of low B-vitamin levels) is by itself toxic to embryos, causing spina bifida and other neural-tube defects. Today the March of Dimes, known for its antipolio campaign of the 1950s, has become a leading advocate of folic acid supplementation before and during pregnancy.

Down Syndrome

Although the role of poor maternal nutrition in the development of Down syndrome has not been delineated, research on other types of birth defects points to its being a critical factor. In addition, the risk of delivering an infant with Down syndrome increases with a woman's age, suggesting that age-related deterioration of a woman's eggs (and the DNA in those eggs) plays a role. In experiments researchers have shown that the DNA of people with Down syndrome is more susceptible to free-radical damage and is not efficient at repairing itself.

Childhood Brain Cancer
See page 166.

What You Can Do

Researchers from the Centers for Disease Control recently reported that folic acid or a multivitamin supplement containing folic acid, taken by a pregnant woman, reduces her risk of delivering a child with any type of birth defect.

Cleft Lip and Cleft Palate

In her above-mentioned study, Steegers-Theunissen found that women who consumed large amounts of folic acid from foods (such as leafy green vegetables) or supplements had a relatively low risk of bearing children with a cleft lip or a cleft palate. This lower risk was evident in women with either MTHFR gene polymorphisms or a normal MTHFR gene. In a separate study, Scottish and Brazilian researchers found that women who took vitamin supplements had about a 40 percent lower risk of delivering children with either a cleft lip or a cleft palate.

As a general rule, if you are of childbearing age, take a moderately high-potency multivitamin supplement with 400 mcg of folic acid. If you have already given birth to a child with a cleft lip or a cleft palate and plan to become pregnant again, take a multivitamin supplement and increase your total folic acid intake to 1,000 to 2,000 mcg day. If you were born with a cleft lip or a cleft palate, ask your physician to measure your homocysteine levels; the birth defect may increase your B-vitamin requirements.

Spina Bifida

Researchers have clearly demonstrated that folic acid supplements (400 to 800 mcg daily) or multivitamins containing folic acid can significantly reduce a woman's risk of delivering an infant with spina bifida or other neural-tube defects. The timing of supplementation is critical. The neural tube forms and closes between the seventeenth and thirtieth days after conception (or four to six weeks after a woman's last menstrual period)—which is usually before many women realize they are pregnant. Taking supplements after this time will not reduce the risk of birth defects. For this reason the March of Dimes, the U.S. Public Health Service (USPHS), and other organizations recommend that all women of childbearing age take a daily multivitamin that contains 400 mcg of folic acid.

If you already have had a pregnancy affected by spina bifida (or other neural-tube defect, the USPHS recommends that you take 400 mcg of folic acid daily if you are *not* planning to become pregnant. However, if you have delivered an infant with spina bifida and you *do* plan to become pregnant again, the USPHS recommends that you take 4,000 mcg of folic acid daily starting at least one month before trying to become pregnant.

Lest we ignore the overall diet, a study published in the *American Journal of Clinical Nutrition* reported that women who ate large amounts of dietary sugars (such as sucrose and high-fructose corn syrup), other highly refined carbohydrates, and potatoes had a higher risk of delivering infants with spina bifida and other neural-tube defects. Such a diet is typically low in B vitamins, quality protein, and vegetables.

Down Syndrome

In the 1950s Dr. Henry Turkel began developing a regimen for treating some of the genetic consequences of Down syndrome. His program, which grew out of his earlier work on genetics and biochemistry, consisted of giving patients with Down syndrome moderately high levels of vitamins and minerals, plus some prescription drugs (such as thyroid medication). Turkel found that the combination of vitamins, minerals, and medications could offset many of the disastrous consequences of Down syndrome. While his nutrition-medication program cannot alter the genetic cause of Down syndrome, it did appear to improve overall gene function and biochemistry.

Turkel found that the earlier a child began receiving supplements, the more normal his or her intelligence and appearance would be by the mid- to late teens. Although Turkel had been recognized for his role in developing lifesaving medical equipment during World War II, his work with Down syndrome was largely ignored by medical organizations. Many people have continued recommending nutritional programs similar to Turkel's, including Bernard Rimland, Ph.D., the director of the Autism Research Institute in San Diego ([619] 281-7165 or www.autism.com/ari/), and Kent MacLeod, B.Sc. Pharm., of Nutri-Chem in Ottawa, Ontario ([613] 820-9065 or www.nutrichem.com).

Recent research on nutrition and Down syndrome appears consistent with Turkel's findings. Dr. Bruce A. Yankner of the Harvard Medical School has reported that brain cells in children with Down syndrome produce three to four times more free radicals, compared with normal children. These free radicals likely exacerbate damage to brain-cell DNA, interfere with cognitive development, and contribute to the increased the risk of Alzheimer's disease.

Yankner reported that antioxidants, including vitamin E and N-acetylcysteine, could, in test tubes, prevent the destruction of brain cells obtained from children with Down syndrome. Meanwhile, researchers at the University of Chile have reported that vitamin E can reduce chromosome damage in lymphocytes obtained from people with Down syndrome. Subsequent research by Yankner indicated that impaired mitochrondrial function was also involved in Down syndrome. That finding suggests that supplemental alpha-lipoic acid, coenzyme Q10, and carnitine might also be helpful. (See "Fatigue and Chronic Fatigue Syndrome" later in this chapter.)

CHILDHOOD BRAIN CANCER

Dr. Susan Preston-Martin of the University of Southern California at Los Angeles led a team of international researchers who investigated the relationship between maternal use of multivitamins during pregnancy and the subsequent risk of brain cancer in children. Her study focused on 1,051 children with brain cancer and 1,919 healthy children. She found that pregnant women who took multivitamin supplements were, overall, 40 percent less likely to have children who developed brain cancer. However, women who took vitamins for the greatest length of time had children with the lowest risk of brain cancer.

Cancer

What Happens

All normal cells have clear biological functions and a cycle of life, beginning when they are created. When cells malfunction or get old, this life cycle ends with apoptosis, a type of biologically programmed self-destruction. In contrast, cancer cells do not have a normal biological function, and they do not have the built-in failsafe of apoptosis. Cancer cells grow uncontrollably, destroying organs and draining the body's nutritional resources for energy, normal growth, and healing.

All cancers result from some type of alteration in DNA that modifies how a gene functions. Although certain genetic traits and types of damage (discussed in the next section) may increase the risk of some types of cancer, the disease more often arises from random damage to DNA, combined with or followed by a massive failure of the body's innate cancer-surveillance and -control systems. In essence, cancers develop as a result of a complex interplay of genetics, diet, lifestyle, and environmental factors. And for as much as we do understand about the origins of cancer, there is much that we do not understand.

Researchers have found that tracing an inherited risk of cancer can be a vexing process. The reason is that people often "inherit" (or adopt) the eating and lifestyle habits of their parents, which are powerful influences on the risk of developing cancer. Hundreds, if not thousands, of factors can come into play in causing a cancer. For example, tobacco smoke is a well-known carcinogen, but not every smoker develops cancer. The reason is that some people, for genetic reasons, are far better than others at breaking down and disposing of toxins. Diet interacts with these factors—some foods, such as cruciferous vegetables, contain vitamin-like substances that enhance the body's ability to detoxify and neutralize tobacco smoke, smog, alcohol, pesticides, and other hazardous chemicals.

Most cancer-causing mutations form in one of two ways. One results from free-radical damage to DNA, which accumulates with age and also explains why the risk of cancer increases with age. The other results from nutritional deficiencies, particularly of folic acid and other B vitamins, which are needed for DNA production and repair and for maintaining overall genetic stability. The effect of an outright deficiency of one or more B vitamins, which may affect 10 to 20 percent of Americans, is comparable to being exposed to radiation from a nuclear bomb. DNA literally breaks apart, preventing genes from functioning normally. Furthermore, a lack of B vitamins, as discussed in chapter 5, prevents the normal suppression of cancer-causing oncogenes.

Aside from their random damage to DNA throughout the body, free radicals and nutrient deficiencies also increase the likelihood of mutations in genes specifically related to cancer risk. Once cancers form, their growth can be promoted by emotional factors and hormones. Cancers also generate large numbers of their own free radicals, creating a condition that spawns further mutations in cancer cells, often making at least some of them resistant to conventional medical chemotherapy and radiation therapy.

The Gene Connection

TUMOR-SUPPRESSION GENES

Researchers have so far identified an estimated seventeen hundred oncogenes—that is, genes that appear to be involved in initiating or promoting cancer growth. These genes, as well as cancer-causing mutations in DNA, are suppressed through a variety of mechanisms. One of these mechanisms is DNA methylation, which depends on folic acid and other B vitamins.

Several genes have been identified as having specific cancer-suppressing roles. Of these the p53 gene (which programs protein 53) is the best understood. The p53 gene plays a key role in inhibiting cancer-cell growth, but the gene can become ineffective when it is mutated. Defective p53 genes have been identified in more than fifty types of cancer—including about 30 percent of breast cancers, 50 percent of brain cancers, and 90 percent of cervical cancers. In rare cases defective nonfunctioning p53 genes are inherited, leading to an increased risk of cancer among most members of the same family. Folic acid and selenium help maintain the normal activity and genetic stability of p53.

Meanwhile, the GST gene codes for several types of glutathione-S-transferases, enzymes that play important roles in preventing cancer. Glutathione-S-transferases function as antioxidants that protect against free-radical damage, and they also aid the body's breakdown of hazardous chemicals. However, researchers have estimated that half of white and about one-third of African Americans in the United States have defective versions of the GST gene. In one study, researchers found that the GST gene was absent in four out of five women with gliomas, a type of brain cancer. Polymorphisms in the GST gene have also been linked to inflammatory diseases and allergic reactions to air pollutants, such as diesel exhaust.

Vitamin D Receptor (VDR) Gene

The VDR gene codes for the vitamin D receptor, which influences how efficiently the body uses vitamin D. Researchers have identified a variety of VDR polymorphisms, and some polymorphisms have been strongly associated with an increased risk of breast, prostate, and colon cancer. Considerable pharmaceutical research is under way to develop synthetic vitamin D molecules that might be effective anti-cancer drugs. (See further discussion of the VDR gene in "The Vitamin D Quandary" section of this chapter.)

Breast and Cervical Cancers

In a typical year, approximately 200,000 women in the United States will be diagnosed with breast cancer, and about 45,000 will die from it. Despite exhaustive research, only a handful of genes have been linked to an increased risk of breast or cervical cancers. The risk associated with these genes must be seen in the proper context: while having one of these genes increases a woman's lifetime risk of breast cancer, not every woman with the gene will in fact develop breast cancer.

Of these genes, BRCA1 and BRCA2 are the best known and most studied. However, assessing the risk posed by the BRCA1 and BRCA2 genes is a little like entering a statistical jungle. In the United States, one or both of these genes are found in fewer than 0.5 percent of women overall but are found in about 2.5 percent of Jewish women of Eastern European heritage. Although BRCA1 and BRCA2 are commonly described as breast-cancer genes, they normally serve important functions in lactation and cancer-cell suppression. Normal turns to abnormal when the BRCA1 or BRCA2 genes are mutated, and there is evidence that these genes are inherently unstable and prone to damage. Having mutations in BRCA1 and BRCA2 genes increases a woman's risk of breast cancer by 60 to 85 percent and cervical cancer by 15 to 40 percent. In the end, mutations in these genes account for only about 2 percent of all breast cancers.

Researchers also believe that the CHEK2 gene is associated with an increased risk of breast cancer. CHEK2 is involved in recognizing and repairing DNA damage and preventing cancer. However, mutations in the CHEK2 gene have been identified in 4.2 percent of women diagnosed with breast cancer and who also had a strong family predisposition of developing the disease. While the CHEK2 mutation modestly increases the risk of breast cancer in women, men with the mutated gene have a tenfold greater risk of developing breast cancer.

Again, the vast majority of breast-cancer cases have not been associated with any specific type of genetic mutation or defect.

PROSTATE CANCER

Some 189,000 men in the United States are diagnosed with prostate cancer, and 30,000 die from the disease each year. While several genes have been associated with prostate cancer, the links are not particularly strong. Rather, certain dietary and lifestyle factors increase the risk of genetic damage in prostate cells, setting the stage for prostate cancer.

The hereditary prostate-cancer gene (HPC1) has been studied the most, although its association with prostate cancer has not been consistent. Several other genes involved in the metabolism of male hormones have also been associated with prostate cancer, but none seems to play a dominant role.

Rather, as in cancer in general, it appears that a variety of mutations, accumulating over several decades, increase the risk of prostate cancer. These mutations are likely the result of chronic prostate infection or inflammation, such as prostatitis, which generates large numbers of free radicals. The risk is compounded by a diet low in protective antioxidants and high in fat. Indeed, research has consistently shown that consumption of antioxidant-rich vegetables and fruits lowers the risk of prostate cancer, whereas diets high in red meats and fats increase the risk.

What You Can Do

Medical testing for the presence of some cancer-associated genes is available, but it is expensive. For example, genetic testing for BRCA1 and BRCA2 costs about three thousand dollars, though some insurers will cover this cost if a woman has a strong family risk of developing breast cancer. However, bear in mind that the absence of these genes may provide a false sense of security about having a low likelihood of developing breast or cervical cancer.

DIET

Your best chance of reducing your risk of cancer is through a combination of diet, supplements, and lifestyle. Hundreds of scientific studies have shown that people eating diets high in vegetables and fruits have a relatively low risk of most cancers. Follow the dietary guidelines described in chapter 7, with an emphasis on nonstarchy vegetables, fruit, fish, and culinary herbs. Herbs are rich sources of a wide variety of antioxidants, and garlic, as an example, has been shown to protect DNA from damage.

SELENIUM

Selenium forms part of several glutathione peroxidase compounds, among the body's most powerful antioxidants. If you do not obtain adequate dietary selenium, your body will not be able to make these antioxidants. Like other antioxidants, these glutathione peroxidases help prevent free-radical damage to genes, which can increase the risk of cancer.

In a landmark study of 1,300 men and women, people who took 200 mcg of selenium daily for an average of four and a half years benefited from significant reductions in the risk of several cancers. Selenium supplements lowered the risk of prostate cancer by 63 percent, colorectal cancer by 58 percent, and lung cancer by 46 percent, according to a report in the *Journal of the American Medical Association*. A separate study, conducted at the Fred Hutchinson Cancer Research Center in Seattle, found that patients with high blood levels of selenium had about half the risk of developing precancerous cell changes in the esophagus.

VITAMIN E

In a review of fifty-nine studies on vitamin supplements and cancer risk, Ruth E. Patterson, Ph.D., of the University of Washington found that vitamin E was most consistently linked to a low cancer risk. In one study, relatively small amounts of supplemental vitamin E (50 IU daily) lowered the risk of prostate cancer by 48 percent over a nine-year period.

In cell and rodent research, the natural succinate form of vitamin E (d-alpha tocopheryl) appears to have potent anticancer effects, far beyond those of other forms of vitamin E. It works in part by inducing apoptosis (self-destruction) of cancer cells, but it does not harm normal cells. Kedar N. Prasad, Ph.D., of the University of Colorado has reported that vitamin E succinate inhibits the growth of many different types of cancer cells, including those of the breast, prostate, colon, and skin. Research has also shown that vitamin E succinate enhances the effects of radiation, chemotherapy, and hyperthermia in killing cancer cells.

FOLIC ACID

This B vitamin, along with vitamins B_6 and B_{12}, helps maintain normal DNA-repair processes and suppresses the activity of cancer-promoting oncogenes. Low levels of these nutrients lead to "genome instability" and increase the risk of cancer.

COENZYME Q10

Women with breast cancer and noncancerous breast lesions commonly have low blood levels of coenzyme Q10, a vitamin-like nutrient. Although CoQ10 functions as a protective antioxidant, its anticancer properties seem more related to boosting the activity of immune cells to fight cancer.

In several journal articles, Dr. Knud Lockwood reported the use of high doses of CoQ10 (390 mg daily) to prevent the recurrence of breast cancer in women. Lower dosages did not provide consistent benefits. CoQ10 may have particularly important functions in the prevention of breast cancer, although this has not yet been studied.

LYCOPENE

In the mid-1990s Dr. Edward Giovannucci of Harvard University reported that men eating ten or more weekly servings of tomato sauces were 45 percent less likely to develop prostate cancer. Tomatoes are rich in lycopene, a potent antioxidant that concentrates in the prostate. A later report by Giovannucci described fifty-seven human studies in which tomatoes were associated with a lower risk of lung, breast, esophagus, and colon cancers.

Relatively few studies have been conducted on pure lycopene, and the research suggests that the active components consist of lycopene *and* other carotenoids found in whole tomatoes and sauces. These other carotenoids include phytoene, gamma-carotene, neurosporiene, phytofluene, beta-carotene, and zeta-carotene.

In a recent study, Dr. Omer Kucuk of Wayne State University in Detroit used a lycopene-rich tomato extract to significantly reduce the size of prostate cancer tumors. He asked 15 men with recently diagnosed prostate cancers to take a tomato extract (containing 30 mg of lycopene, plus other tomato antioxidants) daily for three weeks before surgery. After surgery the prostates of these men were compared with those of 11 men who did not receive supplements before surgery. Lycopene reduced the size of the men's tumors and blocked the cancer's invasive metastasis of other tissues. Eighty percent of the men taking lycopene supplements had relatively small tumors, compared with fewer than half of the men not receiving the supplements. In addition, 73 percent of men taking lycopene had tumors confined to the prostate, compared with only 18 percent of the nonsupplemented group.

COMBINING ANTIOXIDANTS WITH CHEMOTHERAPY

Some nutritionally oriented physicians have also used large dosages of vitamins and minerals to treat cancers, often in conjunction with or after conventional medical therapies. Dr. Jeanne Drisko of the University of Kansas Medical Center has successfully treated cases of cervical cancer with daily dosages of vitamin E (1,200 IU), coenzyme Q10 (300 mg), vitamin C (9 grams), beta-carotene and mixed carotenoids (25 mg), and vitamin A (10,000 IU). The regimen includes intravenous vitamin C (60 grams twice weekly), as well as conventional chemotherapy. These nutrients do not directly affect tumors. Rather they boost the ability of the body's many different immune cells to attack the cancers.

As you might imagine, many other factors influence the growth of cancers. High levels of some hormones, such as estrogen (estradiol), testosterone, and insulin are known to promote cancer growth. Living in cities with significant air pollution, using tobacco products, and drinking excessive amounts of alcohol also increase the risk of cancer—mainly by increasing free-radical mutations to DNA. In addition, certain chronic emotional states, such as depression, can increase the risk of cancer, mostly likely because of underlying alterations in DNA methylation.

Cardiovascular Diseases

What Happens

Coronary artery (heart) disease is the leading cause of death among Americans and other Westerners. Stroke, a type of cardiovascular disease affecting blood vessels in the brain, is the third leading cause of death. Each year in the United States, approximately 700,000 people die from heart disease and 160,000 die from stroke.

In general, coronary heart disease is characterized by an abnormal thickening of the inner walls of arteries within the heart, which reduces blood flow. The heart, like every other organ, depends on a steady supply of oxygen and nutrients, which are delivered via the bloodstream. An interruption of blood flow to the heart causes what is popularly known as a heart attack. The most common type of stroke, called an ischemic stroke, follows a similar pattern in that it is caused by a blockage in a blood vessel that interrupts blood flow to the brain. Hemorrhagic strokes, a less common type of stroke, result from the rupture of a blood vessel in the brain.

The Gene Connection

Researchers have identified several specific genetic variations that can predispose people to cardiovascular disease. However, the risk posed by these genes can almost always be offset through healthier eating patterns and lifestyle habits. Furthermore, it appears that most cases of cardiovascular disease result from more generalized and extensive damage to genes and nongene cell structures, which ultimately impair normal heart function. While much of this damage is age-related—that is, acquired slowly over many years—the rate of gene damage to heart cells can be slowed significantly.

People who inherit one or two copies of genes (from one or both parents) that program for an inefficient form of methylenetetrahydrofolate reductase (MTHFR), an enzyme essential for folic acid utilization, have an increased risk of suffering a heart attack or ischemic stroke. This defect is technically known as the MTHRF 677 C→T genotype. Although it can be tested for, it is usually far easier simply to measure blood levels of homocysteine and then to interpret the results with a physician.

Elevated homocysteine levels, a recognized risk factor for heart disease and stroke, directly damage cells forming blood vessel walls, setting in motion a series of events leading to the deposition of cholesterol. Homocysteine is also a sign of poor methylation, suggesting that the body's production and regulation of DNA activity is impaired. An extremely high homocysteine level indicates that you are not properly utilizing folic acid, because of either low dietary intake or a genetic polymorphism. Either way the remedy is the same: eating more leafy green vegetables (rich in folic acid) and taking a high-potency B-complex vitamin supplement.

Some people have variations in a gene that programs one of the body's cholesterol-transporting proteins. For example, people with an inefficient APOE E4 variation of the apoliprotein gene, which is relatively common in some parts of Scandinavia, tend to have higher blood-cholesterol levels and are more likely to suffer a heart attack. In contrast, the APOE E2 variation of the gene, common in Japan, programs for a very efficient form of apoliprotein, which helps maintain low levels of cholesterol and reduces the risk of a heart attack.

Another important factor comes into play with cholesterol, and that is the susceptibility of low-density lipoprotein (LDL) to free-radical-induced oxidation. Such oxidation is more likely to occur when people consume large amounts of polyunsaturated fats (found in most cooking oils and fried foods), which increase vitamin E requirements.

Oxidized LDL, but not normal LDL, triggers an inflammatory immune response known to be an early step in the development of heart disease. During this immune response, white blood cells seek out and capture oxidized LDL globules, and then the LDL-loaded white blood cells become lodged in blood vessels, where they release free radicals and damage the blood vessel walls. These free radicals circulate in heart cells, causing genetic damage and accelerating the aging of heart cells.

Some people suffer from familial hypercholesterolemia, an inherited condition that causes extreme elevations of cholesterol and other blood fats and a greater risk of premature coronary artery disease. Many studies have found that supplemental vitamins E and C, or the addition of plant sterols (plant extracts found in supplements and some margarines), can lower cholesterol levels in children and adults with familial hypercholesterolemia and, presumably, reduce their long-term risk of heart disease.

A study published in the January 1, 2004, issue of the *New England Journal of Medicine* shed further light on the role of genetic defects and inflammation in heart disease. James H. Dwyer, Ph.D., of the University of Southern California in Los Angeles and his colleagues investigated specific genetic polymorphisms, signs of heart disease, and measures of inflammation in 470 middle-aged men and women. Dwyer focused specifically on polymorphisms in the ALOX5 gene programming for 5-lipoxygenase, an enzyme involved in the body's production of inflammation-promoting molecules.

Genetic testing found that 6 percent of the subjects had polymorphisms in the ALOX5 gene, and these variations were associated with two signs of heart disease: a narrowing of the internal diameter of blood vessels and a doubling of C-reactive protein levels, an indication of low-grade inflammation in the heart. However, the polymorphisms in the ALOX5 gene did not by themselves lead to heart disease. Rather the subjects' diets strongly influenced their risk. People whose diets were rich in linoleic acid (found in corn, safflower, and other common cooking oils) and arachidonic acid (made in the body from linoleic acid) were far more likely to have signs of heart disease. In contrast, people who consumed more omega-3 fats, found in fresh (nonbreaded, nonfried) fish, did not have signs of heart disease.

What You Can Do

From a dietary standpoint, emphasize nutrient-dense foods, particularly wild, cold-water fish and fresh, steamed, or stir-fried vegetables. Recent research has confirmed that reducing dietary carbohydrates—starches and sugars—is far more effective than avoiding saturated fat in improving cardiovascular risk factors. If you avoid vegetables, you risk increasing your homocysteine levels.

B Vitamins

An ideal homocysteine level is less than 6 micromoles per liter of blood. As homocysteine levels increase, so does your risk of heart attack and stroke, and homocysteine levels above 13 mmol/L indicate a serious risk. In most people homocysteine levels can be decreased by taking 400 to 800 mcg of folic acid daily. However, it is better to take a high-potency B-complex or multivitamin supplement that includes at least 50 mg of vitamin B_6 and 100 mcg of vitamin B_{12}. Although elevated homocysteine levels are usually directly linked to folic acid levels, inadequate amounts of these other B vitamins can also result in excess homocysteine.

Vitamin E

Some research has shown that the deleterious effect of the APOE E4 gene can be prevented with vitamin E. In addition, vitamin E helps prevent the oxidation of LDL, which is a more serious problem than moderately elevated LDL or total cholesterol. Unfortunately, LDL oxidation is rarely measured outside of university research settings. For most people 200 to 400 IU of vitamin E daily should be sufficient. If you have elevated LDL or total cholesterol, consider supplementing with 400 to 800 IU. With higher cholesterol levels, your vitamin E levels increase because you need more relative to the greater amount of cholesterol. Also, if you have made a habit of eating a lot of fried foods (burgers, fried chicken, french fries), the extra vitamin E will help reduce oxidation from the consumption of fried oils. Supplemental vitamin C (1,000 mg) daily will also be beneficial.

Selecting a vitamin E product can be confusing. Natural vitamin E is absorbed into the blood and tissues twice as efficiently as are synthetic forms. Therefore it makes sense to purchase natural-source vitamin E. Natural vitamin E will be identified in fine print on the label as d-alpha tocopherol, d-alpha tocopheryl acetate, or d-alpha tocopheryl succinate. (Synthetic is identified as dl-alpha.) Some natural vitamin E products include other types of vitamin E molecules, such as mixed tocopherols and tocotrienols. The natural d-alpha form provides the lion's share of vitamin E's antioxidant properties, but the other forms may also be worthwhile.

Other antioxidants, such as vitamin C and coenzyme Q10, have also been shown to reduce LDL oxidation. Several studies have shown strong relationships between vitamin C intake and longevity, as well as a lower risk of stroke. Vitamin C is essential for the body's manufacture of heart cells and for maintaining the structure and flexibility of blood vessels.

FATTY ACIDS

In my earlier book, *The Inflammation Syndrome*, I detailed the relationship between inflammation and heart disease. Over the past few years, medicine has largely recognized heart disease as an inflammatory disorder of blood levels. As confirmed by the above-mentioned study on the ALOX5 gene, some nutrients have a decidedly proinflammatory effect on heart disease, arthritis, allergies, and many other diseases. Processed foods, rich in common cooking oils and refined carbohydrates, provide excessive quantities of the nutrients involved in the body's inflammatory response. In contrast, omega-3 fish oils, in either cold-water fish (such as salmon, herring, and tuna) or supplements, have a decidedly antiinflammatory effect. Other nutrients, such as gamma-linolenic acid (found in borage, evening primrose, or black currant seed supplements), oleic acid (found in olive oil), and antioxidants also enhance the body's native antiinflammatory processes.

Your individual risk of cardiovascular diseases is also the result of a great many factors besides diet, which ultimately help maintain normal gene function or cause gene damage. Smoking tobacco products generates large quantities of free radicals, which damage the heart, lungs, and other organs. Antioxidant supplements can reduce some of the damage, but not all of it. Being overweight increases the risk of heart disease, as do chronic psychological stress and a sedentary lifestyle. Each of these risk factors—even those with a genetic basis—are modifiable.

Cardiomyopathy and Heart Failure

What Happens

The heart is a muscle, and cardiomyopathy is a weakening of this muscle, which reduces the heart's ability to pump blood. Cardiomyopathy is different from the more common coronary artery disease, in which a narrowing of blood vessel walls reduces the flow of blood within the heart.

Idiopathic dilated cardiomyopathy is characterized by an enlargement and thinning of the heart muscle, which reduces heart function. It accounts for about 80 percent of all cardiomyopathy cases. Hypertrophic cardiomyopathy results from a thickening and stiffening of the heart muscle, which reduces heart function. It accounts for about 20 percent of all cardiomyopathy cases. Heart failure, in which the heart cannot pump sufficient blood to nourish the body with oxygen and nutrients, can result from either cardiomyopathy or coronary artery disease.

The Gene Connection

The heart, which beats approximately a hundred thousand times daily, has enormous energy requirements. Healthy heart cells are rich in mitochondria and the energy-promoting nutrients described in chapter 4, including coenzyme Q10, alpha-lipoic acid, and carnitine. While cardiomyopathy can result from rare inherited genetic defects, it is more commonly the result of acquired genetic damage or a severe depletion of mitochondrial nutrients without genetic damage.

In some cases viral infections lead to myocarditis, an inflammation of the heart muscle. Such viral infections can disrupt the DNA in heart cells and lead to the deaths of large numbers of heart cells. Melinda Beck, Ph.D., of the University of North Carolina at Chapel Hill and Orville Levander, Ph.D., of the U.S. Department of Agriculture have shown that infection with the coxsackie virus, a common cause of sore throats and coldlike symptoms, combined with selenium deficiency, can lead to a viral infection of the heart and heart failure.

Heart failure can also be induced by cholesterol-lowering "statin" drugs, including atorvastatin, lovastatin, prevastatin, and simvastatin. Statins inhibit a key enzyme involved in the body's production of cholesterol. However, the same enzyme is also necessary for the body's production of coenzyme Q10, a vitamin-like substance that plays a crucial role in producing energy in heart cells. So when statin drugs block the body's production of cholesterol, they also reduce the production of CoQ10.

What You Can Do

Age-related damage to mitochondrial DNA can be a cause of cardiomyopathy and heart failure. However, in many cases cardiomyopathy and heart failure stem from an extreme depletion of energy-promoting nutrients. This depletion can be the result of diets high in refined and processed foods, which fail to provide crucial nutrients or the building blocks of those nutrients.

CoQ10

Also known as ubiquinone, CoQ10 is found in every cell of the body, though people with cardiomyopathy and heart failure typically have low levels of it. It is not surprising that replenishing CoQ10 improves heart function in these patients. In one typical study, researchers used CoQ10 supplements to treat 11 heart failure patients who were likely candidates for transplant surgery. All of the patients improved, some regaining normal heart function without any other medications. More recently, in *Molecular Aspects of Medicine*, Dr. Peter Langsjoen reported 200 mg of CoQ10 daily helpful in the treatment of hypertrophic cardiomyopathy, which is characterized by a thickening and stiffening of the heart muscle. Therapeutic amounts typically range from 240 to 360 mg daily in divided doses.

Carnitine

A component of protein, carnitine helps transport fats into mitochondria, where they are burned for energy. It also regulates the use of coenzyme A, an energy-producing compound built around the B vitamin pantothenic acid. Dr. Ioannis Rizos of the University of Athens Medical School studied 70 patients who took either 2 grams of carnitine or a placebo daily for three years. The patients suffered from heart failure resulting from dilated cardiomyopathy. Those who took carnitine had a much better rate of survival compared with those taking the placebo. Over the course of the three-year study, 6 of the patients taking the placebo died, whereas all but 1 of the patients taking carnitine survived. In addition, only 1 patient in the carnitine group developed arrhythmias, compared with 7 in the placebo group. Try 2 grams daily in divided doses.

Vitamin B_1

Patients with heart failure are commonly deficient in vitamin B_1 (thiamine), needed for several key energy-producing chemical reactions. This deficiency can be exacerbated with diuretic drugs used to treat symptoms of heart failure. Several studies have found that vitamin B_1 can improve heart function in patients with heart failure. For example, Dr. David Ezra of the Sheba Medical Center in Israel reported that both oral supplements and intravenous vitamin B_1

corrected deficiencies induced by the drug furosemide (used to treat heart failure) and improved the pumping action of the patients' hearts. Try 100 to 200 mg daily in divided doses.

Celiac Disease

What Happens

Celiac disease is an inherited intolerance of gluten, a family of related proteins found in wheat, rye, barley, and many other grains. In the disease's most recognized form, gluten proteins trigger an autoimmune response that attacks the intestinal wall. As the surface of the intestinal wall decays, digestion becomes impaired, and the resulting malnutrition frequently leads to anemia and osteoporosis. However, celiac disease often progresses for many years without obvious symptoms, or without physicians' linking symptoms to it.

This deterioration of the digestive tract sometimes leads to "leaky gut syndrome," in which undigested proteins enter the bloodstream and trigger a variety of symptoms resembling food allergies. Other common symptoms of celiac disease include bloating, diarrhea, dermatitis, fatigue, and migraine headaches. In fact, researchers have reported that celiac disease may be intertwined in approximately 250 diseases, including depression, dermatitis herpetiformus, treatment-resistant iron-deficiency anemia, Down syndrome, irritable bowel syndrome, lactose intolerance, multiple vitamin and mineral deficiencies, hypothyroidism, and schizophrenia.

Recent studies have found that celiac disease has been widely under-diagnosed. Because it can cause so many different symptoms, some researchers have referred to it as a "clinical chameleon." By new estimates it may affect approximately one in a hundred Americans and Northern Europeans. Some researchers have estimated that a more generalized form of gluten intolerance, without all the intestinal symptoms of classic celiac disease, may affect almost one-half of the population.

Unfortunately, the estimated prevalence of celiac disease and non-celiac gluten intolerance is confounded by two factors. First, many people who carry the genes for celiac disease do not develop any signs or symptoms of the disease, which suggests that other unidentified genes or environmental factors may be involved. Second, people without a genetic predisposition for gluten intolerance may develop symptoms of celiac disease. The latter situation might be partly explained by the presence of another family of proteins, called lectins, found in wheat and many other grains, which can also trigger abnormal autoimmune reactions. For example, lectin sensitivity has been found in some causes of rheumatoid arthritis.

The Gene Connection

Celiac disease and other forms of gluten intolerance serve as good illustrations of how genes and diet interact. Many thousands of years ago, the HLA-DQ2 and HLA-DQ8 genes, which predispose a person toward celiac disease, were relatively common among humans. During most of human evolution, these genes posed no disadvantage, because people rarely if ever consumed grains. This situation changed approximately ten thousand years ago, when people began cultivating gluten-containing grains.

Once the widespread consumption of gluten-containing grains become common, the incidence of many diseases skyrocketed. The result was that the HLA-DQ2 and HLA-DQ8 genes were being turned on, as were abnormal immune responses. Archaeological evidence from about ten thousand years ago indicates significant postgluten increases in birth defects, osteoporosis, arthritis, rickets, dental enamel defects, infertility, child mortality, and disease and death at all ages. The reductions in fertility and increases in childhood mortality served to reduce the numbers of people carrying the HLA-DQ2 and HLA-DQ8 genes.

Today genetic testing can identify the presence of the HLA-DQ2 gene, which is found in 90 to 95 percent of celiac patients, and the HLA-DQ8 gene, found in 5 to 10 percent of cases. In addition, your physician or gastroenterologist can draw blood to test for IgG and IgA antigliadin antibodies, a worthwhile initial screening for celiac disease. More specific tests for gluten sensitivity include the antitissue transglutaminase (anti-tTG) and IgA antiendomysial tests. A stool test for gluten sensitivity is available, and intestinal biopsies can reveal the extent of intestinal damage from years of eating gluten-containing grains.

A study published in the February 2004 issue of the *Journal of Pediatric Gastroenterology and Nutrition* significantly expanded our understanding of the genetic implications of celiac disease. A team of researchers found that genetic damage decreased when children with celiac disease began eating a gluten-free diet. After two years on a gluten-free diet, children with celiac disease showed levels of genetic damage not significantly greater than that in healthy children. The researchers theorized that the "genomic instability" in untreated celiac disease was a consequence of chronic intestinal inflammation.

What You Can Do

Celiac disease and more generalized gluten intolerance represent a widespread genetic incompatibility with commonly consumed gluten-containing grains. The irony is that they are the principal source of dietary carbohydrates in the United States, Europe, South America, and many other parts of the world.

There are no drugs to treat celiac disease and gluten sensitivity. Rather, the treatment is entirely dietary. Like it or not, people with celiac disease must avoid all gluten-containing foods for the rest of their lives. Complete avoidance of gluten is particularly important in cases of "silent" celiac disease, in which the damage is primarily to the intestine and the consequences (such as osteoporosis) may not be obvious for many years. People with celiac disease must not eat breads, hamburger buns, cereals, pastas, muffins, cookies, pizza, or any fish or chicken dredged in wheat flour. Furthermore, they must learn to become careful readers of food labels for the mention—or mere hint—of a gluten-containing grain. It may be worthwhile as well to avoid dairy products, because lactose intolerance and sensitivity to casein (a protein found in dairy products) is often associated with gluten intolerance.

Because of the dietary restrictions, many people diagnosed with celiac disease become resentful or depressed when they cannot continue to consume processed foods, fast foods, or junk foods with abandon—and suffer the same risk of obesity and diabetes as the rest of the population. Some gluten-free substitutes, such as rice-based breads or pastas, are available at health food stores, but these provide mostly empty carbohydrate calories. In fact, people with celiac disease often come to believe that any gluten-free food is good to eat. However, "gluten-free" often means "nutrient-free," as in the case of gluten-free but highly refined breads, pastas, and cookies.

Other than relieving symptoms of celiac disease, gluten-free carbohydrates are no better than gluten-containing carbohydrates for your overall health. Because they tend to consist of highly refined carbohydrates (often from potato or rice) and sugars, they can increase the risk of obesity, Syndrome X, diabetes, and heart disease. A much more sensible and nutritionally sound approach would be to limit carbohydrate intake while focusing on wholesome, nutrient-dense foods, such as chicken, turkey, fish, and nonstarchy vegetables and fruits. This approach would be consistent with our ancient pregrain dietary habits—and with the recommendations in this book.

Depression and Moodiness

What Happens

Depression and moody behavior, including a tendency toward irritability and anger, have a combination of psychosocial and nutritional roots. In some people the triggering event could be the end of a relationship, the death of a loved one, or working at a stressful job, all situations that can profoundly influence eating habits, normal biochemistry, and gene expression in brain cells. Conversely, certain genetic traits and nutritional and biochemical imbalances can increase a person's susceptibility to depression and moodiness.

Depression, which affects about 20 million Americans in varying degrees, is usually characterized by a profound sense of sadness and hopelessness—the belief that life will not get better. Mild to moderate depression can be treated with both natural and pharmaceutical methods, whereas severe depression is typically very resistant to any treatment. More common "everyday" mood disorders, such as "down" days, irritability, impatience, anger, and hostility, affect millions of people to varying degrees.

The Gene Connection

Some genetic polymorphisms do increase the risk of depression and mood disorders. However, the impact of these polymorphisms depends on diet and stressful events.

As you read in chapter 5, polymorphisms in the gene coding for methylenetetrahydrofolate reductase (MTHFR) reduce the efficiency of folic acid metabolism, leading to inefficient methylation, elevated levels of homocysteine, and impaired DNA synthesis and repair. Polymorphisms in the MTHFR gene also boost a person's risk of depression. The reason is that methylation, which depends on folic acid, vitamin B_6, and other nutrients, feeds into the body's production of neurotransmitters, such as serotonin and taurine. Researchers have found that middle-aged women with elevated homocysteine levels, a sign of poor methylation, are twice as likely to be depressed, compared with women who have normal homocysteine levels.

In addition, polymorphisms in the gene that programs a serotonin-transport protein can also influence susceptibility to depression. One version of the gene codes for a very efficient serotonin transporter, whereas the other codes for a poor transporter. People with the inefficient serotonin-transporter gene are far more likely to experience prolonged depression after a stressful event.

Similarly, people who are genetically predisposed to make and excrete a chemical known as kryptopyrrole are stress-intolerant and highly susceptible to depression, fatigue, lethargy, and schizophrenia. (See "Pyroluria" in this chapter.) Kryptopyrrole binds to vitamin B$_6$ and zinc, resulting in increased excretion of these nutrients, and behavioral manifestations of this double deficiency are common.

What You Can Do

DIETARY CONSIDERATIONS

Low blood sugar—more accurately described as rapid and unpredictable drops in blood-glucose levels—can impair cognitive function and alter moods, increasing feelings of impatience, irritability, anger, and hostility. You might think that eating sugary foods would be the fastest way to elevate blood-glucose levels, but the opposite is true. Sugary foods and refined carbohydrates, which the body quickly breaks down into glucose, briefly raise glucose levels and improve moods. But the surge in glucose triggers the secretion of insulin, which overcompensates in decreasing glucose levels, continuing a vicious cycle.

Foods high in protein (chicken, turkey, fish, lean meats) or fiber (nonstarchy vegetables) stabilize glucose and insulin levels. The benefits are swift. Eating a low-glycemic breakfast—that is, a breakfast that causes a minimal increase in glucose and insulin—will stabilize blood glucose up to lunchtime, providing you do not indulge in a high-sugar midmorning snack.

B VITAMINS

According to David Benton, Ph.D., of the University of Wales, the earliest signs of nutritional deficiencies, presuming one pays attention, are behavioral. In his research Benton has found that vitamin B$_1$ and a high-potency multivitamin produce striking improvements in mood among otherwise healthy young adults. Additional research has shown that folic acid and vitamins B$_6$ and B$_{12}$ increase MTHFR activity, leading to higher production of neurotransmitters and improvements in depression, premenstrual anxiety, and irritability.

St. John's Wort

Several clinical studies have found that St. John's wort is as effective as Prozac and Zoloft in treating mild to moderate depression. The herb also causes fewer side effects than the drugs. In addition, St. John's wort also boosts the liver's detoxification processes, which has advantages and disadvantages. The herb helps the body break down toxic chemicals, such as pollutants, but it also speeds the body's breakdown of many medications, requiring an adjustment in the drug's dosage. If you currently take an antidepressant medication, work with your physician in changing its dosage and that of any other medications you take. A general dosage recommendation for St. John's wort is 300 mg three times daily.

5-HTP

A form of the essential amino acid tryptophan, 5-hydroxy-tryptophan is the chemical precursor to serotonin. Researchers believe that it increases serotonin levels in the brain, which reduces depression and anxiety. A beneficial dosage is 300 to 400 mg daily.

Fatigue and Chronic Fatigue Syndrome

What Happens

Chronic fatigue syndrome (CFS)—so severe that many people suffering from it have difficulty getting out of bed—affects an estimated 2 million Americans. However, more generalized chronic fatigue and tiredness, which may affect one-fourth of adult Americans, is the most common physical complaint physicians hear from their patients. Both conditions are characterized by persistent tiredness, but CFS is far more severe and often includes extreme muscle weakness, feelings of depression, and mental fuzziness.

The Gene Connection

Chronic fatigue syndrome is often precipitated by a flulike infection or a significant exposure to pesticides. The feeling of being "wiped out" does not go away. The Epstein-Barr virus (which also causes mononucleosis) is frequently a cofactor in CFS. All viruses are capable of disabling and rewriting DNA, and it is conceivable that severe viral infections disrupt the genes governing cellular energy production. A more speculative theory, but a plausible one, holds that pesticides can poison some of the biochemical pathways involved in energy production.

(Similarly, cyanide kills by almost immediately shutting down mitochondrial activity throughout the body.) Depression is often intertwined in CFS, and it may be the principal symptom of CFS. Feelings of depression can help sustain fatigue, weakness, and lethargy.

More general chronic fatigue and tiredness (in contrast to CFS) can have a variety of causes apart from damaged mitochondrial DNA. Diets high in sugars and refined carbohydrates, bouts of hypoglycemia, prediabetes and diabetes, low thyroid activity, obesity, psychological stress, inadequate sleep, and depression can be interconnected with fatigue. In some cases excess copper levels can depress zinc and result in fatigue.

What You Can Do

Physicians often use energy-promoting nutrients, such as alpha-lipoic acid, B vitamins, carnitine, and coenzyme Q10, to treat mitochondrial myopathies. These same nutrients are often helpful in treating CFS and chronic fatigue, because they provide the nutritional underpinnings of biochemicals involved in energy production. Most of these nutrients are discussed in chapter 4 and elsewhere in chapter 10, so they will be reviewed only briefly here.

Alpha-Lipoic Acid

Alpha-lipoic acid, a vitamin-like nutrient, works in two principal ways. It improves the efficiency of insulin, enabling the body to burn more blood sugar for energy. It also accelerates the energy-producing biochemical reactions within mitochondria, leading to higher ATP levels in the body and the brain. Dosage: 50 to 300 mg daily.

B Vitamins

Vitamins B_1, B_2, and B_3 play crucial roles in breaking down glucose and fat for energy. High intake of carbohydrates increases requirements for vitamin B_1 (needed to make enzymes involved in breaking down carbohydrates) and very likely those of the other B vitamins. Patients with CFS have been shown to have low levels of vitamins B_1, B_2, and especially vitamin B_6.

Although technically not a B vitamin, NADH (nicotinamide adenine dinucleotide) is built around vitamin B_3 and plays a central role in cellular energy production. In a study conducted at Georgetown University Medical School, Dr. Joseph Bellanti reported that 10 mg of NADH daily led to gradual improvements in CFS patients.

CARNITINE

Carnitine helps transport fats into mitochondria, where they are burned for energy. In a study of 28 men and women with CFS, Dr. Audius V. Plioplys of Mercy Hospital and Medical Center in Chicago reported that 3,000 mg of carnitine daily for eight weeks led to significant improvements in symptoms. Inadequate intake of vitamin C, needed for the body's own synthesis of carnitine, can cause fatigue, so vitamin C may be helpful in dosages of 1,000 mg or more daily.

COENZYME Q10

Like the other nutrients discussed in this section, CoQ10 is essential for cellular energy production. Some cardiologists use it to treat cardiomyopathy and heart failure. Dr. Peter Langsjoen has reported that CoQ10 increased energy levels in otherwise healthy octogenarians. Dosages range from 30 to 300 mg daily.

Hemochromatosis

What Happens

Hemochromatosis is the most common genetic cause of iron overload. Although iron is an essential nutrient, high levels can be toxic, though it may take many years for symptoms to become clinically significant.

The disease typically affects people of Northern European heritage and is relatively rare in blacks and Hispanics. More than 1 million Americans have hemochromatosis, and its prevalence in Britain and other Northern European countries may be as high as 1 in every 140 people.

Hemochromatosis leads to the excessive storage of iron in the liver, the endocrine (hormone-producing) glands, and the skin. Diagnosis of the disease is often missed early in life because symptoms, such as arthritis, impotence, fatigue, and low thyroid, may be vague and attributed to other causes. Individual symptoms are often related to the organs in which iron is stored, which impairs the function of those organs. For example, excess iron storage in the liver may lead to cirrhosis or liver cancer, whereas iron storage in the heart may lead to cardiovascular disease. More clear-cut symptoms do not usually appear until after age forty, and these symptoms may also include bronze-colored skin, diabetes, cardiomyopathy, heart failure, and premature death.

The Gene Connection

Hemochromatosis is usually caused by a mutation in the HFE gene. Because of the mutation, the amino acid tyrosine is substituted for cysteine during the production of hemoglobin. This seemingly minor change alters the way the body stores iron. The mutation is referred to as HFE C282Y, because it occurs at position 282 of the HFE gene.

A second gene mutation, H63D, occurs in a small number of hemochromatosis patients. It is likely that other genes besides HFE are involved in iron-storage diseases. Researchers have also identified signs and symptoms of hemochromatosis in people without known genetic markers of the disease, suggesting that either additional genes or lifestyle factors can also lead to iron overload.

In a blood test, elevated levels of iron or serum ferritin levels may be suggestive of hemochromatosis. However, additional testing is required for confirmation.

Some evidence suggests that people with hemochromatosis may have had a survival advantage in ancient times. People with celiac disease commonly suffer from iron deficiency (because of poor absorption), and the HFE mutation may have ensured that people stored sufficient amounts of iron.

What You Can Do

Although it may sound odd, prophylactic phlebotomy—otherwise known as bloodletting—is the standard medical treatment for hemochromatosis. It is an effective way of reducing blood (and subsequently liver) levels of iron. Begun early enough, it can reduce the risk of iron-related disease and premature death, enabling people with the disease to have normal life expectancies.

Some dietary strategies may also be of benefit. In a study of 18 patients with genetically confirmed hemochromatosis, researchers found that regular consumption of black tea with meals significantly reduced iron storage as well as the frequency of bloodletting. The need for bloodletting might also be reduced by avoiding processed, iron-fortified foods, including breads and pastas, and iron-containing vitamin and mineral supplements. Some companies, such as Thorne Research (www.thorne.com), market iron-free supplements. In addition, iron from vegetables is absorbed less efficiently than is iron from meat.

Inflammatory Diseases

What Happens

Nearly everyone is familiar with the redness, swelling, and pain associated with inflammation. Inflammation is a normal process that helps our bodies fight infections and also initiates healing after an injury. After that healing, the inflammatory response should subside. In chronic inflammatory diseases, however, the inflammatory reaction continues and becomes destructive.

Common inflammatory diseases include rheumatoid arthritis, osteoarthritis, allergies, and asthma. Increasing research indicates that most and perhaps all diseases involve excessive inflammation. For example, coronary artery disease is now considered an inflammatory disorder of blood vessels, and high levels of inflammation have been identified in Alzheimer's disease, cancer, diabetes, obesity, and many other diseases.

The Gene Connection

During an inflammatory response, several key transcription proteins, such as nuclear factor kappa-beta and tumor necrosis factor, turn on numerous genes involved in inflammation. Some of these genes code for cytokines, such as interleukin-6 (IL-6) and C-reactive protein (CRP), which signal other immune cells to amplify the inflammatory response.

At the same time, various types of white blood cells become activated. These white blood cells use free radicals to destroy bacteria, virus-infected cells, or damaged cells. Some of these free radicals stimulate genes that program various types of adhesion molecules, which enable white blood cells to stick to normal cells, again sustaining an inflammatory reaction. The cytokines, particularly IL-6 and CRP, signal cells to increase production of another family of hormonelike proinflammatory molecules, including prostaglandin E2.

Our biology heritage has erred on the side of powerful inflammatory responses, and for good reason. Historically, infections and injuries have been the principal causes of death. As recently as 1900, infections were still the leading cause of death in the United States, and even today they remain the leading cause of death worldwide. To survive, humans needed an aggressive immune response.

But why doesn't this inflammatory response turn off after it is needed? The reason, as I explained in *The Inflammation Syndrome*, is that modern refined and processed foods provide large amounts of the building blocks needed for the body's inflammatory response but relatively few of the nutrients required to moderate inflammatory reactions. Diets rich in the omega-6 family of fats (found in corn oil, safflower oil, and other common cooking oils) contribute to the immune response, such as by increasing the antiinflammatory activity of the ALOX5 gene. In contrast, the omega-3 fats (found in fish, flaxseed, and leafy green vegetables) lessen the inflammatory response. Our ancient diet provided relatively equal and balanced amounts of these fats. Processed and refined foods provide twenty to thirty times more of the proinflammatory omega-6 fats.

In addition, most people eat relatively small amounts of vegetables and fruits, depriving them of antioxidants that also have antiinflammatory benefits. Together, the large amount of omega-6 fats, combined with relatively small quantities of omega-3 fats and antioxidants, set the stage for an unbalanced inflammatory response and chronic inflammatory diseases.

What You Can Do

As you might expect, the composition of your diet influences the activity of genes involved in inflammation. For example, the ALOX5 gene codes for 5-lipoxygenase, an enzyme needed to make inflammation-promoting molecules. However, this gene's activity is regulated in part by the relative amounts of dietary omega-6 and omega-3 fats. In people consuming large amounts of omega-6 fats, the ALOX5 gene produces substantial amounts of 5-lipoxygenase and proinflammatory compounds. But when the diet is rich in omega-3 fats, the gene codes for less 5-lipoxygenase and small amounts of proinflammatory substances.

A nutrient-dense diet can be easily tailored to emphasize a variety of antiinflammatory foods. Cold-water fish, such as wild salmon, is particularly rich in antiinflammatory omega-3 fats, and it can be baked in olive oil, which contains antiinflammatory omega-9 fats. The fish can be served with nonstarchy vegetables, such as cauliflower and broccoli, which contain inflammation-suppressing antioxidants. Such an antiinflammatory diet should avoid or strictly limit consumption of refined carbohydrates and sugars, because these foods lead to increases in CRP.

Several supplements can enhance the antiinflammatory effect of a nutrient-dense diet.

FISH-OIL SUPPLEMENTS

Fish-oil supplements contain substantial amounts of omega-3 fats, specifically eicosapentaenoic acid (EPA) and docosahexaenoic acid (DHA). They reduce levels of prostaglandin E2 and other inflammation-promoting compounds, resulting in lower medication requirements. Omega-3 fish oils, in a range of 1 to 5 grams daily, are particularly helpful in arthritis because they inhibit aggrecanases, a family of enzymes that break down cartilage.

GAMMA-LINOLENIC ACID (GLA)

Although GLA is an omega-6 fat, it behaves more like an antiinflammatory omega-3 fat, and the two are synergistic. Several studies have found that GLA, in dosages of 1.4 to 2.8 grams daily, is particularly helpful in rheumatoid arthritis. Supplement sources include borage, black currant, and evening primrose seed oils. The dosage is far more important than the source.

ANTIOXIDANTS

As a general rule, antioxidants have antiinflammatory properties. Several studies have found that vitamin E can lower IL-6 and CRP levels by as much as 50 percent. Consistent with this antiinflammatory effect, vitamin E can also ease symptoms of rheumatoid arthritis. Other antioxidants, particularly flavonoids, such as Pycnogenol and quercetin, have potent antiinflammatory properties. They work in part by reducing the activity of genes involved in inflammation, including those that program adhesion molecules.

Osteoporosis

What Happens

Osteoporosis refers to a serious reduction in the density of bone, which increases the risk of fractures and falls. According to the National Osteoporosis Foundation, 10 million Americans have osteoporosis, and 18 million more have low bone mass (or low bone-mineral density). Eighty percent of people with osteoporosis are women. Each year osteoporosis accounts for 1.5 million fractures of the hip, wrist, vertebrae, and other bones.

Contrary to popular opinion, bones are not completely solid. Under a microscope they look porous, somewhat like a dry sponge. As bone-mineral density decreases and osteoporosis develops, the natural openings in bone increase in size. With lower mineral density, bones become more likely to break under stress.

Because of advertising by the dairy industry, many people believe that calcium is the only nutrient needed for healthy bones. In truth, your bones are living tissue, consisting of a matrix of calcium, magnesium, other minerals, and protein. Every day your body forms new bone and breaks down old bone. As you get older, particularly if you are a postmenopausal woman, you have to work a little harder to maintain normal bone density.

The Gene Connection

In recent years considerable research has focused on the role of vitamin D in maintaining and increasing bone density. Without vitamin D your body cannot put calcium to work. Yet large numbers of people carry polymorphisms in the vitamin D receptor gene (VDR) that interfere with the body's use of the vitamin. (See "The Vitamin D Quandary" in this chapter.)

Some specific VDR polymorphisms are common in people with osteoporosis. Because these polymorphisms reduce the efficiency of vitamin D metabolism, the consequence is often similar to an outright vitamin D deficiency. With low vitamin D activity, all vitamin D–dependent activities, including calcium utilization, are reduced.

What You Can Do

The effect of VDR polymorphisms can be overcome with increased production or intake of vitamin D. By spending fifteen minutes daily in the sun, you can ensure that your body will make adequate amounts of vitamin D. If you spend most of your time indoors or if you live in a cloudy climate, consider taking 400 to 800 IU of supplemental vitamin D each day.

CALCIUM AND VITAMIN D

Combining calcium and vitamin D supplements can make a big difference in bone health. In a study of 389 elderly men and women, Dr. Bess Dawson-Hughes of Tufts University reported that daily supplements of calcium (500 mg) and vitamin D (700 IU) for three years significantly increased bone density. People taking the supplements had half the fractures of a group taking a placebo.

According to a 1997 report issued by the National Academy of Sciences, most Americans do not consume enough calcium. In that report researchers noted that most people fail to obtain the recommended amounts of calcium (1,000 mg daily for people ages twenty-five to fifty and 1,200 mg daily for people over age fifty-one). Only 10 percent of the elderly receive adequate calcium.

MAGNESIUM

The mineral magnesium is, in importance, second only to calcium in bone, and high calcium intake can suppress magnesium levels. In fact, magnesium deficiency, whatever the cause, contributes to weaker bones. In one study Austrian researchers gave magnesium supplements to 24 men in their twenties and thirties. After a month the men benefited from lower bone turnover, a sign of greater resistance to osteoporosis. A beneficial amount is 300 to 400 mg daily.

VITAMIN K

The body's production of several bone-building proteins, including osteocalcin, requires vitamin K. James Sadowski, Ph.D., and his colleagues at Tufts University gave 9 healthy young men and women 420 mcg of vitamin K daily. After fifteen days tests indicated that the subjects' bone density increased, according to an article in the *American Journal of Clinical Nutrition*. Consider taking 100 to 400 mcg daily, but discuss this supplement with your doctor if you are taking anticoagulant (blood-thinning) medications.

VITAMIN B_{12}

Vitamin B_{12} stimulates the activity of two types of osteoblasts, cells needed for bone formation. Your supplement regimen should include 100 to 500 mcg daily.

VITAMIN C

Proteins are woven into the matrix of minerals in bones, and vitamin C is needed to make these proteins. A study of 1,892 middle-aged women in the Seattle area found that those taking vitamin C supplements for at least ten years had higher bone density than women who did not take supplements. The dosage is not specific but may vary from 500 to 2,000 mg daily.

DIETARY CONSIDERATIONS

Several studies have found that high intake of nonstarchy vegetables is associated with increased bone density. In addition, mineral water provides substantial amounts of calcium and magnesium, and antioxidants in green tea also appear to promote bone density.

WEIGHT-BEARING EXERCISES

Walking, weight lifting, and other exercises that place weight on the bones increase bone density. Even modest levels of physical activity are helpful.

If you have been diagnosed with osteoporosis, ask your physician to test you for celiac disease. (See the "Celiac Disease" section in this chapter.) Grains interfere with calcium absorption, and approximately 3 percent of people with osteoporosis have celiac disease. However, about one-fourth of people with celiac disease have osteoporosis, chiefly because of poor nutrient absorption.

—⁓—

The Vitamin D Quandary

For years dietitians have cautioned about excessive intake of vitamin D supplements. The body can store the vitamin, and chronic excesses are potentially fatal, though toxicity and fatalities are extremely rare. Today a growing concern in medicine is over whether people get *enough* vitamin D. Several large studies have found that vitamin D deficiencies are common, particularly among the elderly and people with osteoporosis.

At last count, researchers have identified fifteen polymorphisms in the vitamin D receptor gene (VDR). This gene programs the construction of the vitamin D receptor in cells, and the VDR is the ultimate arbiter of how well your body uses vitamin D. When the VDR cannot function efficiently, vitamin D activity decreases throughout the body.

VDR polymorphisms are surprisingly common, and they have been identified in people with osteoporosis, periodontal disease, type 2 diabetes, Addison's disease, inflammation, psoriasis, and breast, prostate, and colon cancers. Indeed, the relationship between low vitamin D levels and cancer is so well established that there is widespread research on synthetic forms of vitamin D as chemotherapeutic drugs for the treatment of cancer. Low levels of vitamin D also have been found in people with type 1 diabetes, multiple sclerosis, and congestive heart failure, suggesting that VDR gene polymorphisms may be involved in these diseases as well.

Thousands of years ago, when humans spent much of their time outdoors, VDR polymorphisms were of no serious consequence. Sunlight initiates the conversion of cholesterol in the skin to vitamin D. People make prodigious quantities of vitamin D when exposed to sunlight for just a few minutes (and before they get sunburned). These huge amounts of vitamin D saturate the VDR, enabling it to function at optimal levels, regardless of whether a polymorphism is present.

VDR polymorphisms have become more of a health issue because many people now spend much of their time indoors (at home and at work), or they wear sun-blocking clothing and sunscreen while outdoors. In addition, grain consumption reduces vitamin D absorption. Today many of us have little regular exposure to sunlight—our avoidance often compounded by fears of skin cancer—and relatively few dietary sources of vitamin D.

The vitamin D made by your body is extraordinarily safe—no cases of endogenous vitamin D toxicity have ever been reported. The body regulates its own vitamin D production, shutting it off when levels are adequate. If you don't spend much time in the sun, consider taking 400 to 800 IU of vitamin D daily.

—⁓—

Obesity and Type 2 Diabetes

What Happens

Obesity and type 2 (adult-onset) diabetes are almost always linked. Underlying both of these disorders is insulin resistance, reflecting impaired glucose tolerance and the overconsumption of refined carbohydrates and sugars.

Here's what happens: The starches and sugars in refined and processed foods (such as pastas, breads, sugary soft drinks, muffins, bagels, pastries, and candy bars) are quickly digested, leading to a rapid increase in blood-glucose levels. Elevated glucose triggers the secretion of insulin, the hormone that lowers glucose levels by shuttling it from the blood into cells.

For many years elevated insulin levels (an early sign of diabetes risk) can maintain normal glucose levels. However, at a certain point cells will start to resist (or become insensitive to) the action of insulin. When this happens, both glucose and insulin levels remain abnormally high, increasing the risk of elevated cholesterol and triglyceride levels, hypertension, coronary artery disease, blindness, kidney disease, nerve damage, circulatory problems leading to amputation, Alzheimer's disease, and cancer.

The health problems are not just related to high levels of glucose and insulin. Even small increases in blood-sugar levels, well within the normal range, can significantly boost the risk of diabetes and death from heart disease, according to several recent studies. Furthermore, according to Dr. David S. Ludwig of the Harvard Medical School, regularly eating high-carbohydrate and high-sugar foods creates an up-and-down blood-sugar cycle, leading to frequent bouts of hunger and encouraging the consumption of still more high-calorie foods.

Elevated glucose levels reflect the consumption of excessive carbohydrate calories and, often, a lack of compensatory physical activity to help burn those calories. High levels of glucose start what is essentially a free-radical chain reaction, and these free radicals are responsible for some of the tissue destruction associated with diabetes. However, elevated insulin levels may actually be responsible for far more tissue damage.

The Gene Connection

Some population groups, such as the Pima Indians of southern Arizona, are especially prone to obesity and diabetes. Approximately two-thirds of Pima Indians are obese and one-half have diabetes, suggesting a particularly strong genetic predisposition for these diseases. However, no single "smoking gun" gene has been consistently identified as the cause of obesity or diabetes in any group of people.

Rather, the rapidly increasing worldwide prevalence of obesity and diabetes reflects the abnormal juxtaposition of a modern refined diet on our ancient genes. As traditional populations around the world—for example, Australian aborigines, black Africans, Pacific Islanders, and Yemenite Jews—have adopted Westernized eating habits, their incidences of obesity and diabetes have increased by up to forty times.

The risk of diabetes is lower among people of Northern European heritage, suggesting a delayed response to a diet that promotes obesity and diabetes. (It is possible that ten thousand years of refined-grain consumption in Europeans and the ancestors of Europeans has selected for the survival of people with greater resistance to diabetes.) However, in the United States alone, two-third of adults are now overweight or obese, and the incidence of diabetes increased by 36 percent during the 1990s alone. According to a 2003 report from the Centers for Disease Control and Prevention, one of every three children born in

2000 will likely become diabetic because of poor eating habits and a lack of exercise.

A variety of nutritional, biochemical, and genetic factors are at play in obesity and diabetes. As people consume more refined carbohydrates and sugars, their metabolism increasingly resembles prediabetic patterns of blood glucose and insulin. Elevated glucose levels increase the formation of free radicals and advanced glycation end products, both of which damage DNA and other cell structures. Meanwhile, elevated insulin levels alter normal gene behavior, increasing the number and size of fat cells around the belly, accelerating the development of coronary artery disease, and increasing the risk of breast cancer and other types of cancer.

The situation in the United States has been exacerbated by a significant increase in the number of calories consumed. This trend started about fifteen years ago, with "supersize" and larger "value" meals sold at fast-food restaurants, and it is now being exported to Europe and Asia. Food portion sizes are larger today than they were twenty years ago. When public health authorities recommended low-fat diets (purportedly to reduce the risk of heart disease), food companies responded by making and marketing thousands of low-fat and no-fat foods—but the fat was replaced with refined carbohydrates and sugars.

Diets high in refined carbohydrates and sugars displace more nutritious foods, such as fish, meat, and vegetables. As a consequence, people consume fewer nutrient-dense foods and lower levels of the very nutrients (such as B vitamins, alpha-lipoic acid, carnitine, and vitamin C) needed to break down and burn carbohydrates and sugars for energy. Indeed, a study in the February 12, 2004, issue of the *New England Journal of Medicine* found that defects in mitochondrial activity lead to the accumulation of fat in muscle and greater insulin resistance in patients with type 2 diabetes.

What You Can Do

In most people obesity and diabetes are nutritional diseases, and they are best treated nutritionally. Your first step should be to adopt a nutrient-dense diet, consisting of protein and fiber-rich vegetables (see chapter 7). Protein and fiber help stabilize and lower both blood-glucose and insulin levels. One immediate benefit of such eating habits will be a reduction in hunger pangs, leading to less snacking and overeating and a loss of weight. You may not eliminate a tendency toward obesity or diabetes, but such eating habits will certainly help you avoid these two diseases.

Several supplements have been found helpful in reducing glucose levels and enhancing insulin function. It is far better for your body to use less insulin but to use it more efficiently.

CHROMIUM

Chromium, an essential mineral, is needed for the proper functioning of insulin. Studies by Dr. Malcolm N. McLeod, a psychiatrist at the University of North Carolina School of Medicine, found that chromium picolinate supplements (averaging 400 mcg daily) relieved depression, reduced hunger and appetite, and, in some patients, led to significant weight loss. A separate study by U.S. and Chinese researchers found that 1,000 mcg of chromium picolinate daily reduced glucose and insulin levels to almost normal after four months.

SILYMARIN

This antioxidant extract of milk thistle *(Silybum marianum)*, silymarin is widely used to enhance the function of the liver, which works in tandem with the pancreas to regulate glucose levels. In a twelve-month clinical study, 600 mg daily of silymarin reduced glucose in diabetic patients by 9.5 to 15 percent. The patients also benefited from lower levels of sugar in the urine, less glycated hemoglobin, and lower insulin requirements.

ALPHA-LIPOIC ACID

Like silymarin, alpha-lipoic acid also improves insulin function and lowers blood-sugar levels. It is widely used in Germany to treat diabetic symptoms, including nerve damage. Alpha-lipoic acid helps the body break down and burn glucose for energy, and as an antioxidant it protects against diabetic complications.

In a series of animal experiments described in the journal *Nature Medicine* in 2004, researchers reported that supplemental alpha-lipoic acid reduced appetite and led to both weight and fat loss. According to the researches, alpha-lipoic acid worked by reducing levels of the enzyme AMP-activated protein kinase (AMPK). AMPK levels increase when cell reserves of glucose and fat decrease, and it plays a key role in stimulating hunger. The therapeutic dose of alpha-lipoic acid is 200 mg three times daily.

CINNAMON

Richard A. Anderson, Ph.D., and his colleagues recently treated diabetic subjects with 1, 3, or 6 grams of cinnamon or a placebo daily. (One gram of cinnamon is about one-quarter teaspoon of the ground herb.) Overall, people receiving cinnamon benefited from 18 to 29 percent decreases in fasting glucose levels, 7 to 27 percent declines in cholesterol levels, and 23 to 30 percent reductions in triglyceride levels. In general, larger amounts of cinnamon had greater benefits.

Apple Cider Vinegar

Carol S. Johnston, Ph.D., of Arizona State University, asked three groups of subjects to drink 20 grams of apple cider vinegar before consuming a high-carbohydrate breakfast containing 87 carbohydrate grams from a bagel, butter, and orange juice. The subjects included 11 people with insulin resistance, 10 with type 2 diabetes, and 8 healthy controls. A week later all the subjects were given a placebo drink followed by the same high-carbohydrate breakfast. All of them benefited from smaller increases in glucose and insulin after consuming the apple cider vinegar.

Parkinson's Disease

What Happens

Parkinson's disease is the second most common neurodegenerative disorder after Alzheimer's disease. It affects an estimated 1 million Americans, and about 60,000 new cases are diagnosed each year. Although Parkinson's disease is often diagnosed in people in their forties, the average age of onset is about sixty years.

People in the advanced stages of the disease have a haunting and unsettling look: their torso remains unnaturally rigid, while tremors uncontrollably shake the arms, hands, legs, and jaw. In addition, balance and coordination are impaired, so people with the disease shuffle about slowly and unsteadily.

The Gene Connection

Although several inherited genes are involved in rare forms of Parkinson's disease, no clear genetic predisposition has been identified in the more common forms of the disease. Twenty percent of patients with Parkinson's disease have a close relative with the disease, suggesting a genetic component. However, 80 percent of cases have no obvious inherited risk.

The disease is better understood in biochemical terms. It is characterized by a catastrophic decrease in the brain's production of dopamine, a neurotransmitter. The drug levodopa provides the chemical precursor to dopamine, but its benefits are limited. Brain cells eventually become insensitive to the benefits of levodopa, and the drug can hasten the onset of dementia. About 40 percent of Parkinson patients taking the drug develop dementia within ten years.

Some researchers have long suspected that regular exposure to chemical toxins, especially pesticides, can damage dopamine-producing neurons in a part of the brain known as the substantia nigra. In one recent study, Mark P. Mattson, Ph.D., of the Johns Hopkins University School of Medicine and his colleagues exposed laboratory mice to a chemical known to cause Parkinson-like symptoms in rodents. The mice were also fed diets either rich in or deficient in folic acid, needed for the production of neurotransmitters.

Mattson reported in the *Journal of Neurochemistry* that a lack of folic acid by itself did not result in any Parkinson symptoms. But when folic-acid-deficient animals were also exposed to the chemical, they suffered a 50 to 60 percent decrease in dopamine-producing brain cells and also exhibited Parkinson-like physical symptoms.

There is also tantalizing evidence that Parkinson's disease may sometimes be related in part to a profound decrease in cellular energy production. Low intake or production of coenzyme Q10 reduces cellular energy production, which may result in neurological diseases, including Parkinson's disease and cerebral ataxia.

What You Can Do

COENZYME Q10

A recent clinical trial, reported in the American Medical Association's *Archives of Neurology*, found that large dosages of vitamin-like CoQ10 significantly slowed the progression of Parkinson's disease. In the study, Dr. Clifford W. Shults of the University of California at San Diego and his colleagues treated 80 patients with Parkinson's disease. The patients were divided into four groups, each receiving 300, 600, or 1,200 mg of CoQ10 daily or a placebo for sixteen weeks.

All the patients taking CoQ10 benefited from a slower progression of Parkinson's disease, but those taking 1,200 mg daily had the greatest benefits. They suffered only about half the deterioration of Parkinson symptoms, compared with patients taking a placebo, and they were most likely to maintain their normal daily activities. This study suggests that Parkinson's disease may involve a significant decay in cellular energy production, and Shults did find that CoQ10 did increase the patients' cellular energy levels.

ANTIOXIDANTS

Considerable evidence points to the toxic effects of free radicals in Parkinson's disease, and several studies point to the protective benefits of antioxidants. For example, Dr. Maarten C. de Rijk of Erasmus University Medical School in Rotterdam reported that people who consumed large amounts of dietary vitamin E had about half the risk of developing Parkinson's disease compared with people who consumed little of the nutrient. Similarly, researchers from Harvard Medical School analyzed the dietary habits and risk of Parkinson's disease among 77,000 female nurses and 47,000 male physicians over twelve to fourteen years. Again, people consuming large amounts of vitamin E from foods had a lower risk of developing Parkinson's disease.

DIETARY CONSIDERATIONS

A nutrient-dense diet plan consistent with the recommendations in chapter 7 may also reduce the risk of Parkinson's disease. Dr. Wiebke Hellenbrand of the Otto von Guericke University in Germany analyzed the eating habits of people with Parkinson's disease and found that they consumed large amounts of refined sugars and other carbohydrates, including sweets, desserts, chocolate, cookies, and cakes, compared with healthy subjects. In addition, they ate relatively few raw vegetables and had low intake of beta-carotene and vitamin C. A separate study found that high consumption of dairy foods, with the exception of butter, more than doubled the risk of Parkinson's disease in men.

Pyroluria

What Happens

An estimated 5 percent of otherwise healthy North Americans excrete a chemical known as kryptopyrrole (technically, 2,4, dimethyl-3-ethyl pyrrole). However, kryptopyrrole excretion increases sharply when people experience chronic psychological stress or suffer from mental illness. For example, an estimated 10 percent of stressed people excrete kryptopyrrole, as do 50 percent or more of schizophrenics.

Kryptopyrrole (also known as urinary pyrroles, the mauve factor, and malvaria) appears to be a by-product of the body's stress response. Kryptopyrrole causes most of its biochemical mischief by binding with vitamin B_6 and zinc, which are also excreted, resulting in a deficiency of both nutrients.

Both vitamin B_6 and zinc play myriad roles in health. Vitamin B_6 is required for the body's production of neurotransmitters, such as serotonin and taurine, and the synthesis and repair of DNA. "Zinc fingers" provide structural and functional roles in DNA, and the mineral also plays roles in cognitive functioning and the senses of taste and smell. Psychological stresses place a greater demand on neurotransmitter production, which in turn uses up more vitamin B_6. Excessive stress in people who are genetically predisposed to excrete kryptopyrrole will increase elimination of vitamin B_6 and zinc, amplifyng the health consequences of that stress.

Women are more likely than men to have pyroluria. Regardless of sex, people with pyroluria tend to have a low tolerance for stress, and they are especially sensitive to the effects of psychological stress, such as work and relationship pressures. They also have high levels of internal tension—they're what would often be described as high-strung—and often complain of depression, fatigue, and lethargy. People with pyroluria may say that they don't dream or never remember their dreams. They may also be more susceptible to the effects of excess dietary copper, which can further suppress zinc levels. White spots in fingernails, a sign of zinc deficiency, may also indicate pyroluria.

The Gene Connection

The specific genetic mutation causing pyroluria has not been identified. Rather, pyroluria is inferred based on the presence of kryptopyrrole in the urine. According to the psychiatrist Dr. Abram Hoffer, 25 percent of nonpsychotic psychiatric patients, 50 percent of chronic schizophrenics, and 75 percent of acute (sudden-onset) schizophrenics have kryptopyrrole in their urine. When these patients are successfully treated, their kryptopyrrole levels return to normal.

What You Can Do

Some nutritional medical centers, such as the Bright Spot for Health in Wichita, Kansas, regularly test patients for kryptopyrrole. Normal levels are less than 20 mcg per deciliter of blood.

Having elevated kryptopyrrole levels in the urine increases a person's vitamin B_6 and zinc requirements. Not surprisingly, people who excrete kryptopyrrole will likely benefit from supplemental vitamin B_6 and zinc. Their sensitivity to zinc depletion will also be helped by avoiding major sources of copper, such as using cookware in which copper is in contact with food or living in older houses that may have extensive copper piping. Copper can be leached by acidic foods (such as tomato sauces) and soft water.

If you are sensitive to the effects of stress or are often anxious or depressed, it might be worthwhile to ask a nutritionally oriented physician to measure your kryptopyrrole level. (Many nonnutritional physicians may say they have never heard of such a test.) Alternatively, if you have symptoms consistent with pyroluria, you could simply begin taking a high-potency B-complex supplement, containing at least 100 mg of vitamin B_6, and 25 mg of zinc daily. If your symptoms ease within thirty days, there is a good chance that you are genetically predisposed to excrete kryptopyrrole. It is important to maintain normal B_6 and zinc levels and to consider stress-reduction techniques.

Sickle-Cell Anemia

What Happens

Sickle-cell anemia is an inherited disease that affects hemoglobin, the oxygen- and nutrient-carrying molecule in red blood cells. More than 60,000 Americans of African ancestry, as well as a small number of people of Mediterranean and Middle Eastern heritage, have sickle-cell anemia. Two million other Americans have what physicians call the sickle-cell trait, which increases the risk of developing some sickle-cell anemia symptoms.

Normal red blood cells are disk-shaped and flexible, bending to squeeze through the body's tiniest blood vessels. They also remain viable for about four months. In contrast, sickle cells—so named because of their sickle or crescent shape—break down after only ten to twenty days, causing chronic anemia. Sickle cells also tend to lodge in blood vessels, forming clots that reduce the oxygen supply, cause pain, and increase the risk of cardiovascular diseases. They can also damage the spleen, kidneys, and other organs. Other symptoms include shortness of breath and greater susceptibility to infection.

Thousands of years ago, people with the sickle-cell trait had a survival advantage. Sickle-shaped red blood cells are resistant to the parasite that causes malaria, and people with this trait were more likely to survive malaria epidemics. Today, with malaria eradicated in most of the developed world, the gene responsible for sickle-cell anemia poses far more hazards than benefits.

The Gene Connection

The disease results from an inherited genetic defect, technically known as the HbS mutation, which substitutes the amino acid valine for glutamate during the construction of hemoglobin. This simple change has profound consequences, altering the shape and increasing the stickiness of hemoglobin molecules.

Sickle-cell anemia was the first disease to be recognized as having molecular, or genetic, origins. This discovery was made in 1949 by Nobel laureate Linus Pauling, Ph.D., who later studied the molecular roles of vitamins in heart disease, cancer, schizophrenia, and other diseases.

The HbS mutation causing sickle-cell anemia cannot be changed. However, nutritional supplements can overcome HbS-related anemia and other nutrient deficiencies, restore normal blood levels of nutrients, and reduce many symptoms of the disease. It is very likely that a nutrient-dense diet, emphasizing fish and fresh vegetables, will also improve health and reduce symptoms.

What You Can Do

Researchers have found that several dietary supplements can lessen the symptoms of sickle-cell anemia. For example, people with sickle-cell anemia have elevated blood levels of homocysteine, a sign of defective DNA synthesis and a major risk factor for coronary artery disease, stroke, Alzheimer's disease, and some types of cancer.

Tay S. Kennedy, Ph.D., of the Children's Hospital of Philadelphia measured folic acid and vitamin B_{12} levels in 70 sickle-cell patients, ranging in age from infancy to nineteen years old. More than half of them did not consume enough folic acid from food, and despite daily supplementation of 1,000 mcg of folic acid daily, 15 percent continued to have low blood levels of the vitamin. Although most of the subjects had normal blood levels of vitamin B_{12}, both B_{12} and folic acid levels declined with the subjects' age. Such findings suggest that people with sickle-cell anemia need considerable folic acid.

In a study conducted with sets of twins suffering from sickle-cell anemia at the Philadelphia Biomedical Research Institute, S. Tsuyoshi Ohnishi, Ph.D., found that a combination of several high-potency supplements greatly reduced symptoms. Over six months Ohnishi asked 10 patients to take 6 grams of vitamin C, 1,200 IU of vitamin E, 1,000 mcg of folic acid, and 6 grams of aged garlic extract daily. Meanwhile the subjects' twin siblings took only folic acid. People taking the high-potency vitamins had one-third the number of painful sickle-cell episodes, compared with those taking only folic acid.

Red blood cells from people with sickle-cell anemia are more susceptible to free-radical damage, and low intake of vitamin E may increase the risk of sickle-cell symptoms. Supplemental vitamin E helps protect the membranes of red blood cells against free-radical damage. In addition, frequent blood transfusions may boost iron levels, as might iron-containing supplements, which could lead to further free-radical damage to red blood cells.

A cell study at the Philadelphia Biomedical Research Institute tested the effects of green tea extract and aged garlic extract on sickle-cell dehydration, which exacerbates blood-cell damage and may increase clotting. Epigallocatechin gallate, a major antioxidant component of green tea extract, almost completely inhibited sickle-cell dehydration. The garlic extract reduced dehydration by 30 percent.

Taken together, these studies show that people suffering from sickle-cell anemia risk multiple nutrient deficiencies and often have extremely high vitamin requirements. People with sickle-cell anemia should undergo a comprehensive nutrition workup, including blood tests for vitamin levels. At the very least, a high-potency multivitamin (described earlier in this chapter) should be taken. However, higher dosages may be justified if such a supplement fails to raise blood levels of the vitamins.

Skin Aging and Wrinkles

What Happens

The skin, like every other organ, undergoes an age-related deterioration. But unlike other organs the skin is directly exposed to environmental factors that can accelerate its aging—and make you look older than your biological age. Ultraviolet (UV) rays in sunlight age the skin more than almost any other factor, other than perhaps tobacco smoke. The greater a person's exposure to UV rays, the greater the skin damage—though the seriousness of the damage may not be obvious for two to three decades.

When skin ages, its constituent proteins (such as collagen and elastin) break down, lose their elasticity, become tough, and develop ridges. Fats, which normally give skin much of its flexibility, become stiffer and reduce the flow of nutrients into and waste products out of cells. These destructive processes can be slowed and to some extent reversed, but the damage is best prevented or minimized.

The Gene Connection

Free radicals are generated when UV rays strike water molecules in cells. Some UV wavelengths, such as UV-A, cause damage primarily by generating large numbers of free radicals, which then oxidize DNA, proteins, and fats. Other wavelengths, such as UV-B, cross-link the chemical compounds forming DNA, which in turn degrade the integrity of that DNA. Damage that cannot be repaired leads to either poorer-quality DNA in new skin cells or the wholesale loss of skin cells.

Sunburn is essentially an inflammatory response to UV exposure, but very subtle skin-cell damage can be detected before the skin reddens. Within about fifteen minutes of UV exposure, the amount of hydrogen peroxide, a potent generator of free radicals, increases significantly in skin cells. In addition, levels of several proinflammatory molecules, such as cytokines, also begin to increase in the skin.

After about an hour, cell-signaling molecules called protein kinases boost the activity of AP-1, a transcription factor that turns on several genes involved in breaking down the protein matrix forming skin. Specifically, these genes code for collagenase, metalloproteinase, and other enzymes whose job is to break down proteins. At the same time, AP-1 interferes with the genes normally involved in programming production of collagen, one of the principal skin proteins. Interestingly, one of the genes that codes for metalloproteinase is especially active in smokers, just as it is in people who have been exposed to UV rays.

Research by Lester Packer, Ph.D., professor emeritus at the University of California at Berkeley, has shown that the skin normally contains a large reservoir of antioxidants, which protect against modest exposure to UV rays. These antioxidants can be rapidly depleted by intense or lengthy exposure to UV rays. Antioxidant-rich diets and antioxidant supplements work by tempering the activity of genes activated after UV-ray exposure.

What You Can Do

DIETARY CONSIDERATIONS

A diet rich in nonstarchy vegetables and fruits can increase the reservoir of protective antioxidant vitamins, carotenoids, and flavonoids normally found in your skin. In fact, researchers have found that people eating a healthy diet—one consistent with the recommendations in chapter 7—are less likely to develop wrinkles. Dr. Mark L. Wahlqvist of Monash University in Australia analyzed the diets of 453 elderly people of different ethnic groups. Wahlqvist carefully measured the amount of sun-related damage to the subjects' skin, then looked for dietary patterns related to skin aging.

He found that people who consumed a lot of olive oil, beans, fish, vegetables, and other healthy foods experienced relatively little skin damage. In contrast, those who ate a lot of saturated fat, red meat, processed deli meats, sugary soft drinks, pastries, and potatoes were more likely to suffer premature skin damage.

Vitamins E and C

Dr. Bernadette Eberlein-Konig of the dermatology clinic at the Technical University of Munich measured the responses of 20 men and women to artificial UV light. After giving the subjects 1,000 IU of natural vitamin E and 2,000 mg of vitamin C daily for eight days, Konig found that their resistance to sunburn increased by 20 percent. That resistance to sunburn indicated lower levels of inflammation and less damage to skin cells. In contrast, people taking a placebo became more sensitive to sunburn.

Carotenoids

Wilhelm Stahl, Ph.D., of the Heinrich Heine University in Germany asked 36 men and women to take one of three supplements daily for twelve weeks: 24 mg of beta-carotene (equivalent to 40,000 IU); a mixed-carotenoid supplement containing 8 mg each of beta-carotene, lutein, and lycopene; or a placebo. At the end of the study, tests indicated that both carotenoid supplements improved the subjects' resistance to sunburn.

In another study, conducted at the University of Arizona, Ronald Watson, Ph.D., and his colleagues asked 22 men and women to take natural beta-carotene supplements for almost six months. As the dosage increased from 30 to 90 mg, the subjects' skin became increasingly resistant to sunburn from simulated sunlight.

A separate study identified at least one of the reasons beta-carotene protects against sunburn. Scientists at the University of Bath in England, determined how UV rays activated the HO-1 gene, which helps promote the inflammatory response in skin after sunburn. Beta-carotene, however, suppressed the activity of the HO-1 gene.

PYCNOGENOL

Pycnogenol, a natural complex of antioxidants, derived from French maritime pine trees, has also been shown to increase antioxidant reserves in the skin and build resistance to sunburn. Researchers asked 20 fair-skinned men and women to take Pycnogenol supplements (approximately 75 to 120 mg) daily for eight weeks. After four weeks the subjects were 40 percent more resistant to sunburn, and after eight weeks they were 84 percent more resistant. Pycnogenol works partly by reducing the activity of two genes, calgranulin A and B, involved in skin disorders.

INSIDE-OUTSIDE PROTECTION

Several studies have determined that a combination of beta-carotene supplements, taken orally, and topical sunscreens are more effective than sunscreens alone in protecting against sunburn. Although these studies focused only on beta-carotene supplements, it is likely that a multiple-antioxidant supplement (or a high-potency multivitamin) will work just as well, if not better.

ANTIOXIDANT-RICH LOTIONS

Skin creams and lotions rich in antioxidants, such as vitamin C or the herb chamomile, have been shown to reduce wrinkles and improve overall skin tone. Several studies have found that creams containing vitamin C can reverse some of the damage from "photoaging" (sunlight-induced damage) of the skin. Meanwhile, European researchers have found similar impressive benefits from chamomile-containing creams. One high-quality, reliable brand of chamomile-containing creams and lotions is CamoCare.

PAY ATTENTION TO YOUR TIME IN THE SUN

Common sense dictates that you not spend excess unprotected time in the sun, particularly if you live in hot, sunny regions. If you expect to be in the sun, especially during summer months or at high altitudes, for more than ten to fifteen minutes, apply topical sunscreen (SPF 15 or higher) and wear a hat, long pants, and a long-sleeved shirt. This is especially important if you must be outdoors between 10:00 A.M. and 2:00 P.M., when UV rays are their most intense.

It is beneficial, however, to spend a little time in the sun during early-morning or late-afternoon hours, so your body can make vitamin D. For added protection, take a multivitamin supplement that contains at least some of the antioxidants discussed in this section.

AFTERWORD

We are all familiar with the phrase "knowledge is power." Understanding our options in any situation gives us the opportunity to make the best possible decision. The same idea holds true for your health and risk of disease. Given a variety of options, you can make the best possible decision about your health—or you can squander the opportunity.

One of the ironies we face is that the role of genes in health has often been overstated, whereas the role of nutrition has been greatly undervalued. The medical promise of genetics and gene therapy has attracted billions of dollars in investments. By comparison, nutrition research receives paltry funding and lacks the allure of high-tech medicine. Yet nutrition provides all the basic building blocks of your entire body, and nutrients are essential for normal gene function.

For many years physicians and researchers believed that our genetic traits were fixed. They came to this conclusion based on the idea that if some of our genetic traits, such as the color of our eyes, remained the same throughout life, then all of our other genetic traits must stay the same as well. This view amounts to a form of genetic fatalism, a belief that we cannot change a thing with the genes we inherited from our parents.

But the truth is actually the very opposite. We can and often do modify our risk of disease. An obese person can lose weight and lower his or her risk for diabetes. A person with a family history of heart disease can change his or her diet and lifestyle and lessen his or her chances of suffering a heart attack. Doctors routinely tell us that eating better and exercising will reduce our risk of disease. Only recently, however, have they begun to understand that improvements in health are the result of more than just losing weight or controlling cholesterol levels. Underlying all of these visible improvements in health are more basic changes in gene activity.

The lesson in these examples, and in this book as a whole, is that our genes are not rigid. Rather they constantly respond to the cellular environment around them. This means that you are anything but powerless when it comes to modifying the activity of your genes. Because you control what you put into your mouth, you can also control the activity of your genes.

The simple act of eating, the most natural of all habits, forces us to make choices. Again, we can make the best possible decisions or we can squander the opportunity. We can eat fast foods and convenience foods, which are built primarily on sugars, refined carbohydrates, and unhealthy fats. By doing so we set the stage for abnormal gene activity. Or we can consciously decide to resist unhealthy foods and instead opt for wholesome, nutrient-dense foods, such as fish and vegetables. This approach fosters normal, even optimal, gene activity.

Everything you do in life is a choice, and doing nothing or delaying a decision for another day is a choice as well. In *Feed Your Genes Right*, I have provided an explanation and a plan for enhancing your genes and health. I encourage you to use this information to make the right choices, the ones that build the foundation for a long and healthy life. Knowledge *is* power. Use it wisely to promote good health.

APPENDIX A

Genetic and Nutrition Testing

By now you understand that the health and function of your genes are shaped in large part by your individual dietary and lifestyle habits. You also know that you can protect your genes and enhance their activity with a nutrient-dense diet, nutritional supplements, stress reduction, and other positive lifestyle changes. These are changes you can adopt on your own without any genetic testing. I encourage you to make as many of these changes as possible, just as I have done.

But should you consider genetic testing?

Unfortunately, the answer is currently not as straightforward as I would like. Some medical laboratories provide various degrees of genetic testing. (See the list of laboratories later in this appendix.) When done correctly, such testing can reveal important information about how specific genetic polymorphisms, mutations, and other anomalies might affect your nutritional requirements and long-term health. Unfortunately, many genetic tests remain relatively expensive. Because of this, you and your physician may often do just as well interpreting more common blood tests in terms of their genetic and health implications. The situation will certainly improve. In the next two to five years, genetic testing will likely become more sophisticated, more commonplace, and less expensive.

The Potential Downside of Genetic Testing

Sadly, as genetic testing becomes a more common feature on our medical and social landscape, the risk of genetic discrimination will likely increase. But such genetic discrimination does not have to occur.

I believe that you and I will have a right to obtain genetic testing, assuming that the technology is widely available and of reasonable cost. Knowing of certain genetic risks we face would give us an opportunity to make better dietary, lifestyle, and medical decisions.

But there may be a catch. We live in a society in which insurers of one type or another control the purse strings that pay for medical tests and treatments. Insurers are for-profit businesses, and they seek to earn a profit while minimizing their costs. All too often insurers ration health care or deny coverage instead of fulfilling their social obligation.

The consequence may be a collision between your right to know about genetic risks for disease and an insurer's temptation to discriminate against you. There is a legitimate reason for this concern. Insurers have often appeared arbitrary and unfair in denying approvals or payments for medical care, and it is common for an insurer to deny coverage for a preexisting condition. For example, if you have been diagnosed with diabetes and then change jobs and insurers, your new insurer may refuse to pay for the treatment of your diabetes. Like other businesses, insurers are averse to obvious risks or liabilities.

So what will probably happen when insurers are asked to pay for your genetic testing, as they inevitably will be? Just as insurers currently want to learn your medical history, they will undoubtedly want to know the results of your genetic testing. For all practical purposes, the tradition of patient-physician confidentiality does not exist when it comes to insurers. They want to learn as much as possible to predict the cost of your potential future medical claims. In one potential scenario, if insurers learn that you have a genetic predisposition for a serious disease, they may define it as a "predisease," similar to the current definition of a preexisting condition. With a predisease you may be denied insurance coverage, or your insurance may exclude coverage for the predisease.

However, there are possible alternative scenarios.

A genetic predisposition indicates only risk, not destiny, a key point that is often ignored in discussions of genetics. You and I were born with various types of genetic risks for disease, and we acquire additional genetic damage that increases our risk of age-related diseases. Insurers have had a tendency to see a person's risk of disease as a threat to their future profitability. For example, a slight variation in the MTHFR gene increases a person's risk of heart attack, stroke, Alzheimer's disease, depression, and delivering an infant with birth defects, all very costly medical conditions to treat.

But the risks associated with the MTHFR gene can be offset with good dietary habits (such as eating sufficient leafy green vegetables) or for as little as two cents a day in vitamin supplements, adding up to about seven dollars a year. If insurers are at all shrewd, they will recognize that disease prevention through genetic testing, diet modification, and vitamin supplementation is far more cost-effective than is later treatment with drugs, surgery, and hospitalization. Rather than being used as a tool of genetic discrimination, testing, diet, and supplementation can be a way to reduce long-term medical costs.

If there is to be a more rational approach to our future health care, it may be along these lines: Your physician would test you for various genetic predispositions, as well as for levels of vitamins and other nutrients involved in gene and overall cell function. She would make dietary recommendations, such as eating more fish and vegetables, avoiding french fries and soft drinks, and exercising more. She might also recommend certain vitamin supplements. And she would caution you, if you had no obvious genetic predispositions, that you should not be complacent and take your health for granted.

In the process, medicine would shift a significant portion of its current activities related to the expensive and aggressive treatment of disease to less costly prevention. Under these circumstances insurance companies could earn and save millions of dollars, our society's health-care costs would decrease, and nearly everyone would have an opportunity to be truly healthy.

The Upside of Nutrient Testing

So, a bit more practically, how can a person determine his or her individual nutritional requirements, which are shaped by a combination of genetics and lifestyle? It is currently easy and relatively inexpensive to measure blood levels of vitamins and minerals, though only nutritionally oriented physicians routinely do this with patients.

As an example, on several occasions since 1997, I have undergone testing at the Bright Spot for Health, a nonprofit, nutritionally oriented medical clinic in Wichita, Kansas, to assess my nutrient levels. These tests have helped me improve and fine-tune my eating habits and supplement regimen. I'll offer two personal illustrations from my experience there. Several years ago blood tests found that my levels of vitamin B_1 were relatively low. This was odd, because my dietary intake of the vitamin was high, and I had also been taking 50 mg of it as part of a B-complex supplement. (The daily value, or DV, for vitamin B_1 is a scant 1.2 mg.) Only after taking an additional 250 mg of vitamin B_1 daily (more than 200 times the DV) for many months did my B_1 levels increase to normal.

On another occasion, during a period of extreme personal stress, my right arm became stiff and painful to move for many months. I had been taking 50 mg of vitamin B_6 daily. (The DV for B_6 is only 1.7 mg.) Again, after consulting a physician, the evidence pointed to an inadequate intake of vitamin B_6. However, vitamin B_6 is needed for the body's production of serotonin and other neurotransmitters, which may have been compromised by stress. The pain in my arm did not decrease until after I took 500 mg of B_6 daily (almost 300 times the DV) for several months. It took an entire year for me to regain complete mobility of the arm.

What Some Nutritional, Medical, and Genetic Tests Might Reveal

After reviewing your medical history and discussing your symptoms, a physician will likely order a variety of blood tests. These tests might point to genetic mutations, risk factors for disease, or nutritional deficiencies. These are some of the tests you might undergo:

- *Antioxidant Panel.* This test measures blood levels of various nutrients, including vitamins E and C, beta-carotene, and other nutrients.
- *Antitissue Transglutaminase.* A positive test for anti-tTG indicates gluten intolerance, the cause of celiac disease.
- *Aspartate Aminotransferase.* An extremely sensitive test to assess functional vitamin B_6 levels. It measures the activity of an enzyme dependent on B_6, instead of just measuring the vitamin.
- *BRCA1 and BRCA2.* Mutations in these genes are associated with an increased risk of breast and cervical cancer.
- *C-Reactive Protein.* The "high-sensitivity" CRP test reflects your body's level of inflammation, which is involved in most disease processes. A high-sensitivity CRP level of 3.5 mg/dl indicates a high risk of heart disease. Ideal levels are less than 0.1 mg/dl.
- *Glucose.* An elevated fasting glucose (greater than 90 mg/dl), part of all standard blood tests, may indicate a risk of developing diabetes.
- *Glutathione Reductase.* A sensitive test for vitamin B_2 that measures the activity of a key antioxidant enzyme that depends on the vitamin.
- *HbS Mutation.* This mutation indicates either sickle-cell anemia or the less serious sickle-cell trait.
- *HFE Mutations.* Detection of C282Y and H63D mutations indicates hemochromatosis, an iron-overload disease that increases the risk of diabetes, heart disease, and premature death.
- *HLA-DQ2 and HLA-DQ8.* These tests indicate a genetic predisposition for celiac disease, an intolerance of gluten proteins found in wheat and many other grains.
- *Homocysteine.* Elevated homocysteine levels (especially greater than 13 mmol/L) are indicative of low folic acid, possibly low vitamin B_{12}, and poor methylation reactions. An ideal level is between 4 and 8 mmol/L.
- *Insulin.* An elevated fasting insulin level (greater than 20 mcIU/ml) may indicate prediabetic insulin resistance. In fact, insulin levels may be increased years before blood-glucose levels become elevated. An ideal level is less than 12 McIU/ml.
- *Kryptopyrrole.* The presence of kryptopyrrole in the urine indicates that vitamin B_6 and zinc are being excreted at abnormally high rates. Elevated kryptopyrrole is strongly associated with poor stress responses and an increased risk of mental illness.
- *Lipoprotein (a).* This cholesterol subfraction may be indicative of an inherited risk of heart disease. Lp(a) levels above 20 mg/L point to an

increased risk of cardiovascular disease. The ideal level is less than 15 mg/L.

- *Methylmalonic Acid.* This is a very sensitive test for vitamin B_{12} levels. Rather than directly measuring the B_{12} levels themselves, the test looks at the vitamin's functional impact on methylmalonic acid.
- *MTHFR Polymorphisms.* The presence of polymorphisms in the gene coding for methylenetetrahydrofolate reductase may point to increased nutritional requirements for folic acid and an increased risk of coronary artery disease, stroke, Alzheimer's disease, and depression.
- *Transketolase.* A highly sensitive test for vitamin B_1. It measures the activity of an enzyme influenced by B_1 levels.
- *Vitamin D Receptor Gene.* Polymorphisms in the VDR gene interfere with utilization of vitamin D and may increase the risk of osteoporosis, diabetes, cancer, and multiple sclerosis.

Referral Services for Finding a Nutritionally Oriented Physician

The ideal way to assess your overall health and nutritional status is to work with a nutritionally oriented physician. A physician can order laboratory tests for vitamins, minerals, and other nutrients and help you interpret the results and develop a dietary and supplement plan. The following organizations provide Internet-based referral services.

American College for Advancement in Medicine
www.acam.org
International Society for Orthomolecular Medicine
www.orthomed.org
centre@orthomed.org

American Association of Naturopathic Physicians
www.naturopathic.org

Laboratories for Blood and Genetic Testing

Some laboratories (indicated with an asterisk) are equipped to test for genetic variations that interfere with normal nutrient utilization. However, such testing is relatively new to the marketplace and can be expensive. It may be just as worthwhile to arrange for more standard and less expensive blood testing of nutrient levels. Your first round of tests should establish a baseline, indicating where improvements (in nutrient levels) are needed. Follow-up tests should show whether you have achieved these improvements. Most testing laboratories prefer to work with physicians, but some offer home-testing kits. Your physician may be familiar with other laboratories as well.

Bright Spot for Health
(316) 682-3100
www.brightspot.org

Carolyn Katzin* (represents multiple laboratories)
ckatzin@carolynkatzin.com
www.carolynkatzin.com

Genelex Corporation*
(800) 523-3080
www.genelex.com

Great Smokies Diagnostic Laboratory*
(800) 522-4762
www.greatsmokies-lab.com

Pantox Laboratories
(888) 726-8698
www.pantox.com

Your Future Health
(877) 468-6934
yourfuturehealth.com

APPENDIX B

Resources for Supplements, Foods, and Additional Information

Nutritional Supplements

Thousands of companies sell proprietary brands of vitamins, minerals, and other types of nutritional supplements, resulting in an often confusing array of products and competing claims. The companies listed here are known to the author and have particularly high-quality products.

Abkit, Inc.

Abkit manufactures and distributes a variety of excellent supplements and cosmetic products. Its AlphaBetic is a well-rounded once-a-day supplement for people with glucose intolerance or diabetes. The company's extensive CamoCare line of cosmetics is designed around the venerable antioxidant herb chamomile. For more information call (800) 226-6227 or go to www.abkit.com.

Advanced Physicians' Products

Founded by a nutritionally oriented physician, APP offers an extensive line of high-quality vitamin and mineral supplements. For more information call (800) 220-7687 or go to www.nutritiononline.com.

Bioforce

Bioforce is a venerable Swiss maker of herbal products, with a strong commitment to product consistency and quality. For more information call (877) 232-6060 or go to www.bioforce.com.

J. R. Carlson Laboratories
Carlson Laboratories offers the widest selection of natural vitamin E products, as well as a broad range of other vitamin and mineral supplements. For more information call (800) 323-4141 or go to www.carlsonlabs.com.

Juvenon
Founded by researchers Bruce Ames, Ph.D., and Tory Hagen, Ph.D., Juvenon makes an Energy Formula that provides acetyl-L-carnitine and alpha-lipoic acid, discussed in chapter 4 and elsewhere in the book. For more information call (800) 588-3666 or go to www.juvenon.com.

Nature's Way
Nature's Way's products include many German pharmaceutical-grade herbal supplements. For more information call (801) 489-1500 or go to www.naturesway.com

Nordic Naturals
Nordic Naturals markets a line of high-quality fish-oil capsules, with slight differences in formulation designed to support the joints, the cardiovascular system, and brain function. For more information call (800) 662-2544 or go to www.nordicnaturals.com.

Nutricology/Allergy Research Group
Nutricology/Allergy Research Group is often at the cutting edge of original nutritional supplement formulations. Nutricology is the company's consumer brand, and Allergy Research Group is the company's professional (physician's) brand. For more information call (800) 545-9960 or go to www.nutricology.com.

Nutrition 21
Nutrition 21 is the company behind the popular Chromax brand of chromium picolinate, which is also sold under other, more familiar brand names. In addition, Nutrition 21 also sells Chromax and Diachrome, the latter a chromium picolinate–biotin combination.

Pure Scientific
Pure Scientific markets Advantig brand supplements, which target different aspects of health, including energy and body-mind balance. For more information call (877) 877-4566 or go to www.advantig.net.

Thorne Research
Thorne sells its extensive line of high-quality supplements primarily to physicians, but it also accepts orders from consumers. For more information call (208) 263-1337 or go to www.thorne.com.

Natural Food Grocers

Feed Your Genes Right recommends that you eat nutrient-dense fresh and natural foods. Your best bet for finding meat from range- or grass-fed animals and organic fruits and vegetables is a natural foods grocery store.

Trader Joe's

Trader Joe's is a chain of high-quality specialty retail grocery stores, with many organic, gluten-free, and wholesome products. For more information and the locations of Trader Joe's stores, go to www.traderjoes.com

Wild Oats

Wild Oats, a national chain, emphasizes natural and gourmet foods. Their meat departments offer free-range meats. For more information call (800) 494-WILD or go to www.wildoats.com.

Whole Foods

Like Wild Oats, the emphasis at Whole Foods is on wholesome, natural foods, including free-range meats, organic produce, and a wide variety of other healthful food products. For more information go to www.wholefoods.com

Vitamin Cottage

Vitamin Cottage is a Colorado-based, family-owned group of nineteen natural food stores with markets in Denver and other cities in Colorado, as well as in Albuquerque and Santa Fe, New Mexico. For more information and the locations of Vitamin Cottage stores, call (877) 986-4600 or go to www.vitamincottage.com.

Specialty Foods

CC Pollen

If you exercise regularly and intensely, you may require relatively high-carb energy bars. CC Pollen makes Almond-Date, Cinnamon-Apple, and Peanut-Raisin Buzz Bars, which may be the best-tasting energy bars sold. The principal sweetener in these bars is honey, and they also contain small amounts of bee pollen harvested in southern Arizona. Many health food stores and Web sites sell Buzz Bars. You can also order them directly from CC Pollen by calling (800) 875-0096 or visiting www.ccpollen.com or www.buzzbars.com.

Czimer's Game and Seafood

If you live in the Chicago area, you are lucky enough to be near a longtime purveyor of game meat. Czimer's has been in retail business for more than thirty-five years, selling venison, bear, antelope, and other game meats. It is located at 13136 W. 159th Street, Lockport, IL 60441. For more information call (708) 301-0500. (Many other cities have butchers that specialize in game meats—check your phone book or the Internet for information.)

Earth Song Whole Foods

Earth Song makes several whole-grain snack bars that redefine the meaning of a wholesome sweet. Among the bars are Apple-Walnut and Cranberry-Orange. In addition, Earth Song blends an excellent gluten-free muesli, known as Grandpa's Secret Omega-3 Muesli, which makes for a tasty and quick breakfast (if you take about five minutes to prepare it the night before). For more information call (877) 327-8476 or go to www.earthsongwholefoods.com.

Greatbeef.com

Greatbeef.com is supported by more than a dozen independent family farmers who humanely raise livestock and chicken. Most of the animals are free-range or pasture-fed, so that the meat has a natural balance of fatty acids and less saturated fat than corn-fed beef. Members of Greatbeef.com are located in Arizona, California, Colorado, Iowa, Minnesota, Missouri, Nebraska, Nevada, Oregon, Pennsylvania, Tennessee, Texas, and Virginia. For more information about specific ranchers and how to buy meat from them, go to www.greatbeef.com.

Indian Harvest

Indian Harvest, a mail-order firm, sells a variety specialized rices, including black, purple, red, and green rice. For more information call (800) 294-2433 or go to www.indianharvest.com.

Lotus Foods

Lotus Foods sells a selection of original and tasty rice and rice flour products, including Bhutanese Red Rice and purple Forbidden Rice. The rice flours can be used to dredge fish and chicken, as well as to make gluten-free crepes. For more information call (510) 525-3137 or go to www.lotusfoods.com to place an order or to find recipes.

MacNut Oil (Macadamia Nut Oil)

MacNut Oil, made from Australian macadamia nuts, is rich in oleic acid, the same type of fat that makes olive oil so healthy. MacNut Oil has a slightly nutty flavor and a higher smoke point than olive oil. For information call (866) 462-2688 or go to www.macnutoil.com.

Omega Nutrition

Omega Nutrition produces a broad selection of unrefined, organic, and minimally processed cooking oils, which can be shipped directly to your home. For information call (800) 661-3529 or go to www.omegaflo.com.

Terrapin Ridge

Terrapin Ridge makes and sells an extensive line of tasty sauces, such as Apple Dill and Rosemary, Apricot Honey with Tarragon, and Spicy Chipotle Squeeze, as well as fifteen different mustards. If you are tired of the same old chicken, turkey, or beef, these sauces can add bright new flavors to your meals. For more information call (800) 999-4052 or go to www.terrapinridge.com.

Information on the Role of Nutrition in Birth Defects

Autism Research Institute (Autism, Down syndrome)
San Diego, California
(619) 281-7165
www.autism.com/ari

Nutri-Chem, Inc. (Down syndrome)
Ottawa, Canada
(613) 820-9065
www.nutrichem.com

The Warner House
www.warnerhouse.com

March of Dimes (spina bifida and birth defects)
www.modimes.com

Newsletters, Magazines, Books, and Web Sites

Many publications provide excellent information on diet and supplements, though you may sometimes have to navigate contradictory information or ignore information inconsistent with the *Feed Your Genes Right* diet plan.

Newsletters and Magazines

The Nutrition Reporter

The Nutrition Reporter is a monthly newsletter, produced by the author, that summarizes recent research on vitamins, minerals, and herbs. The annual subscription rate is $26 ($48 CND for Canada, $38 in U.S. funds for all other countries). For a sample issue, send a business-size self-addressed envelope, with postage for two ounces, to *The Nutrition Reporter*, P.O. Box 30246, Tucson, AZ 85751. Sample issues are also available at www.nutritionreporter.com.

Let's Live

Let's Live, a monthly magazine, focuses on how diet, nutrition, and supplements help maintain health and reverse disease. The annual subscription is $15.95. To order call (800) 365-3790.

Alternative Medicine

As the title suggests, *Alternative Medicine* is a consumer-oriented magazine that focuses on alternative and nonconventional approaches to healing, including vitamin supplements, diet, and energy medicine. The annual subscription is $24.95, with payment to *Alternative Medicine*, P.O. Box 1056, Escondido, CA 92033-9871.

GreatLife

   GreatLife magazine is not sold by subscription. Rather, it is provided free at leading health food and natural food stores.

Books

The Inflammation Syndrome: The Complete Nutritional Program to Prevent and Reverse Heart Disease, Arthritis, Diabetes, Allergies, and Asthma, by Jack Challem (John Wiley & Sons, 2003, $14.95). With a diet plan similar to the one in *Feed Your Genes Right,* this book is tailored more to people with chronic inflammatory diseases.

Syndrome X: The Complete Nutritional Program to Prevent and Reverse Insulin Resistance, by Jack Challem, Burton Berkson, M.D., Ph.D., and Melissa Diane Smith (John Wiley & Sons, 2000, $14.95). With a diet program similar to the one in *Feed Your Genes Right,* this book focuses more on preventing diabetes and heart disease, as well as losing weight.

The Paleo Diet, by Loren Cordain, Ph.D. (John Wiley & Sons, 2001, $24.95). Cordain, one of the leading experts on the Paleolithic diet, describes the Paleolithic diet, which can be considered the original *Feed Your Genes Right* dietary plan.

Why Grassfed Is Best! The Surprising Benefits of Grassfed Meat, Eggs, and Dairy Products, by Jo Robinson (Vashon Island Press, 2000, $7.50). This small book (128 pages) is worth every penny. It makes a powerful case for eating grass-fed meats and other foods, most of which are compatible with the *Feed Your Genes Right* dietary plan. Included is a list of sources for meat from free-range and pasture-fed animals. Order it from Vashon Island Press, 29428 129th Avenue SW, Vashon, WA 98070. For more information call (206) 463-4156 during West Coast business hours. You can also order it from www.thestoreforhealthyliving.com. Add $4.50 for shipping and handling.

Going Against the Grain: How Reducing and Avoiding Grains Can Revitalize Your Health, by Melissa Diane Smith (Contemporary Books, 2002, $14.95). This book explores how the cultivation and consumption of grains led to a deterioration in people's health. Smith provides dietary plans for eating low-grain and no-grain diets.

Web Sites

The Official Feed Your Genes Right Web Site
www.feedyourgenesright.com

The Official Anti-Inflammation Diet Plan Web Site
www.inflammationsyndrome.com

The Nutrition Reporter
Dozens of articles on vitamins and minerals.
www.nutritionreporter.com

Medline
The world's largest searchable database of medical journal articles, providing free abstracts (summaries) of more than 8 million articles.
www.ncbi.nlm.nih.gov

Merck Manual
The online edition of your physician's standard medical reference book.
www.merck.com

Nutrient Data Laboratory Food Composition
Type in nearly any food or food product and you instantly get its nutritional breakdown per cup or 100 grams.
www.nal.usda.gov/fnic/foodcomp

Paleo Diet/Recipes
Most of these modern versions of Paleolithic recipes are compatible with the nutrient-dense food guidelines described in chapter 7.
www.panix.com/~paleodiet/list/

Price-Pottenger Foundation
A Web site dedicated to two twentieth-century nutritional pioneers.
www.price-pottenger.org

SELECTED REFERENCES

A complete list of references is available at www.feedyourgenesright.com.

General

CHAPTER 1. YOUR GENES DEPEND ON GOOD NUTRITION

Ames, B. N. "Micronutrient Deficiencies: A Major Cause of DNA Damage." *Annals of the New York Academy of Sciences*, 1999; 889:87–106.

Begley, S. "So Much for Destiny: Even Thoughts Can Turn Genes 'On' and 'Off.'" *Wall Street Journal*, June 21, 2002:B1.

Commoner, B. "Unraveling the DNA Myth." *Harper's*, February 2002:39–48.

Kaput, J. "Diet-Disease Gene Interactions." *Nutrition*, 2004; 20:26–31.

Kaput, J., and R. L. Rodriguez. "Nutritional Genomics: The Next Frontier in the Post-genomic Era. *Physiological Genomics*, 2004; 16:166–77.

Kim, Y. I. "Methylenetetrahydrofolate Reductase Polymorphisms, Folate, and Cancer Risk: A Paradigm of Gene-Nutrient Interactions in Carcinogenesis." *Nutrition Reviews*, 2000; 58:205–17.

Moore, D. S. *The Dependent Gene: The Fallacy of Nature vs. Nurture.* New York: Henry Holt and Company, 2002.

Santarelli, L., M. Saxe, C. Gross, et al. "Requirement of Hippocampal Neurogenesis for the Behavioral Effects of Antidepressants." *Science*, 2003; 301:805–9.

Turkel, H., and I. Nusbaum. *Medical Treatment of Down Syndrome and Genetic Diseases.* Southfield, Mich: Ubiotica, 1985.

Van Ommen B., and R. Stierum. "Nutrigenomics: Exploiting Systems Biology in the Nutrition and Health Arena." *Current Opinion in Biotechnology*, 2002; 13:517–21.

CHAPTER 2. DNA DAMAGE, AGING, AND DISEASE

Ames, B. N., H. Elson Schwab, and E. A. Silver. "High-Dose Vitamin Therapy Stimulates Variant Enzymes with Decreased Coenzyme Binding Affinity (Increased Km): Relevance to Genetic Disease and Polymorphisms." *American Journal of Clinical Nutrition*, 2002; 75:616–58.

Arpa, J., A. Cruz-Martinez, Y. Campos, M. Gutierrez-Molina, et al. "Prevalence and Progression of Mitochondrial Diseases: A Study of 50 Patients." *Muscle and Nerve*, 2003; 28:690–95.

Blount, B. C., M. M. Mack, C. M. Wehr, et al. "Folate Deficiency Causes Uracil Misincorporation into Human DNA and Chromosome Breakage: Implications for Cancer and Neuronal Damage." *Proceedings of the National Academy of Sciences*, 1997; 94:3290–95.

Culotta, E., and D. E. Koshland Jr. "DNA Repair Works Its Way to the Top." *Science*, 1994; 266(5193):1926–29.

DiMauro, S. "Exercise Intolerance and the Mitochondrial Respiratory Chain." *Italian Journal of Neurological Science*, 1999; 20:387–93.

Dwyer, J. H., H. Allayee, K. M. Dwyer, et al. "Arachidonate 5-lipoxygenase Promoter Genotype, Dietary Arachidonic Acid, and Atherosclerosis." *New England Journal of Medicine*, 2004; 350:29–37.

Everson, R. B., C. M. Mehr, G. L. Erexson, et al. "Association of Marginal Folate Depletion with Increased Human Chromosomal Damage in Vivo: Demonstration by Analysis of Micronucleated Erythrocytes." *Journal of the National Cancer Institute*, 1988; 80:525–29.

Harman, D. "Free Radical Theory of Aging." *Mutation Research*, 1992; 275:257–66.

Helzlsouer, K. J., E. L. Harris, R. Parshad, et al. "DNA Repair Proficiency: Potential Susceptibility Factor for Breast Cancer." *Journal of the National Cancer Institute*, 1996; 88:754–55.

Hoffer, A., and L. Pauling. "Hardin Jones Biostatistical Analysis of Mortality Data for a Second Set of Cohorts of Cancer Patients with a Large Fraction Surviving at the Termination of the Study and a Comparison of Survival Times of Cancer Patients Receiving Large Regular Oral Doses of Vitamin C and Other Nutrients with Similar Patients Not Receiving These Doses." *Journal of Orthomolecular Medicine*, 1993; 8:157–67.

Jackson, M. J., A. McArdle, and F. McArdle. "Antioxidant Micronutrients and Gene Expression." *Proceedings of the Nutrition Society*, 1998; 57:301–5.

Kopsidas, G., S. A. Kovalenko, J. M. Kelso, et al. "An Age-Associated Correlation between Cellular Bioenergy Decline and mtDNA Rearrangements in Human Skeletal Muscle. *Mutation Research*, 1998; 421:27–36.

Koshland, D. E. "Molecule of the Year: The DNA Repair Enzyme." *Science*, 1994; 266:1925.

Kovalenko, S. A., G. Kopsidas, J. Kelso, et al. "Tissue-Specific Distribution of Multiple Mitochondrial DNA Rearrangements during Human Aging." *Annals of the New York Academy of Sciences*, 1998; 854:171–81.

Lau, N. C., and D. P. Bartel. "Censors of the Genome." *Scientific American*, August 2003:34–41.

Linnane, A. W., S. Kovalenko, and E. B. Gingold. "The Universality of Bioenergetic Disease. Age-Associated Cellular Bioenergetic Degradation and Amelioration Therapy." *Annals of the New York Academy of Sciences*, 1998; 854:202–13.

Miller, G. D., and S. M. Groziak. "Diet and Gene Interactions." *Journal of the American College of Nutrition*, 1997; 16:293–95.

Muller, M., and S. Kersten. "Nutrigenomics: Goals and Strategies." *Nature Reviews/Genetics*, 2003; 4:315–22.

Oltean, S., and R. Banerjee. "Nutritional Modulation of Gene Expression and Homocysteine Utilization by Vitamin B_{12}." *Journal of Biological Chemistry*, 2003; 278:20778–84.

Sancar, A. "Mechanisms of DNA Excision Repair." *Science*, 1994; 266(5193):1954–56.

Sapolsky, R. M. *Why Zebras Don't Get Ulcers: A Guide to Stress, Stress-Related Diseases, and Coping.* New York: W. H. Freeman and Company, 1994.

Sen, C. K., and L. Packer. "Antioxidant and Redox Regulation of Gene Transcription." *FASEB Journal*, 1996; 10:709–20.

Seppa, N. "Metal's Mayhem. Cadmium Mimics Estrogen's Effects, Thwarts DNA Repair." *Science News*, July 19, 2003:38.

Trayhurn, P. "Nutritional Genomics—Nutrigenomics." *British Journal of Nutrition*, 2003; 89:1–2.

Zingg, J. M., and P. A. Jones. "Genetic and Epigenetic Aspects of DNA Methylation on Genome Expression, Evolution, Mutation and Carcinogenesis." *Carcinogenesis*, 1997; 18:869–82.

CHAPTER 3. CONFLICTS BETWEEN ANCIENT GENES AND MODERN FOODS

Ames, B. N., and P. Wakimoto. "Are Vitamin and Mineral Deficiencies a Major Cancer Risk?" *National Review of Cancer*, 2002; 2:694–704.

Baschetti, R. "Genetically Unknown Foods or Thrifty Genes?" *American Journal of Clinical Nutrition*, 1999; 70:420–25.

Burke, W. "Genetic Testing." *New England Journal of Medicine*, 202; 347:1867–75.

Challem, J. J. "Did the Loss of Endogenous Ascorbate Propel the Evolution of Anthropoidea and Homo Sapiens?" *Medical Hypotheses*, 1997; 48:387–92.

Cordain, L., J. B. Miller, S. B. Eaton, et al. "Plant-Animal Subsistence Ratios and Macronutrient Energy Estimates in Worldwide Hunter-Gatherer Diets." *American Journal of Clinical Nutrition*, 2000; 71:682–92.

Dhahbi, J. M., J. H. Kim, P. L. Mote, et al. "Temporal Linkage between the Phenotypic and Genomic Responses to Calorie Restriction." *Proceedings of the National Academy of Sciences*; electronic publication March 22, 2004, ahead of print.

Eaton, S. B., and S. B. Eaton II. "Paleolithic vs. Modern Diets—Selected Pathophysical Implications." *European Journal of Nutrition*, 2000; 39:67–70.

Hursting, S. D., J. A. Lavigne, D. Berrigan, et al. "Calorie Restriction, Aging, and Cancer Prevention: Mechanisms of Action and Applicability to Humans." *Annual Review of Medicine*, 2003; 54:131–52.

Johnston, C. S., and L. L. Thompson. "Vitamin C Status of an Outpatient Population." *Journal of the American College of Nutrition*, 1998; 17:366–70.

Kaati, G., L. O. Bygren, and S. Edvinsson. "Cardiovascular and Diabetes Mortality Determined by Nutrition during Parents' and Grandparents' Slow Growth Period." *European Journal of Human Genetics*, 2002; 10:682–88.

Kiecolt-Glaser, J. K., K. J. Preacher, R. C. MacCallum, et al. "Chronic Stress and Age-Related Increases in the Proinflammatory Cytokine IL-6." *Proceedings of the National Academy of Sciences*, 2003 (early online edition):1531903100.

Lander, H. M. "An Essential Role for Free Radicals and Derived Species in Signal Transduction." *FASEB Journal*, 1997; 11:118–24.

Lev-Ran, A. "Mitogenic Factors Accelerate Later-Age Diseases: Insulin as a Paradigm." *Mechanisms of Aging and Development*, 1998; 102:95–113.

Mattison, J. A., M. A. Lane, G. S. Roth, et al. "Calorie Restriction in Rhesus Monkeys." *Experimental Gerontology*, 2003; 38:35–46.

Pauling, L. "Orthomolecular Medicine." *Science*, 1968; 160:265–71.

Waterland, R. A., and R. L. Jirtle. "Transposable Elements: Targets for Early Nutrition Effects on Epigenetic Gene Regulation." *Molecular and Cellular Biology*, 2003; 23:5293–5300.

Williams, W. J. *Biochemical Individuality: The Basis for the Genetotrophic Concept.* New York: John Wiley & Sons, 1956.

Wright, J. D., J. Kennedy Stephenson, C. Y. Wang, et al. "Trends in Intake of Energy and Macronutrients—United States, 1971–2000." *Morbidity and Mortality Weekly Report,* February 6, 2004; 53:80–82.

CHAPTER 4. NUTRIENTS THAT ENHANCE ENERGY
AND PREVENT DNA DAMAGE

Barbiroli, B., R. Medori, H. J. Tritschler, et al. "Lipoic (Thioctic) Acid Increases Brain Energy Availability and Skeletal Muscle Performance As Shown by in Vivo 31P-MRS in a Patient with Mitochondrial Cytopathy." *Journal of Neurology,* 1995; 242:472–77.

Barbiroli, B., et al. "Thioctic Acid Stimulates Muscle ATP Production in Patients with Type-2-Diabetes and Diabetic Polyneuropathy." *Diabetes und Stoffweschsel,* 1996; 5(Supplement-Heft 3):71–76.

Campos, Y., et al. "Plastma Carnitine Insufficiency and Effectiveness of L-Carnitine Therapy in Patients with Mitochondrial Myopathy." *Muscle and Nerve,* 1993; 16:150–53.

Folkers, K., T. Hanioka, L. J. Xia, J. T. McRee Jr., and P. Langsjoen. "Coenzyme Q10 Increases T4/T8 Ratios of Lymphocytes in Ordinary Subjects and Relevance to Patients Having the AIDS Related Complex." *Biochemical and Biophysical Research Communications,* 1991; 176(2):786–91.

———, and R. Simonsen. "Two Successful Double-Blind Trials with Coenzyme Q10 (Vitamin Q10) on Muscular Dystrophies and Neurogenic Atrophies." *Biocheimica et Biophysica Acta,* 1995; 1271:281–86.

Forsyth, L. M., H. G. Preuss, A. L. MacDowell, et al. "Therapeutic Effects of Oral NADH on the Symptoms of Patients with Chronic Fatigue Syndrome." *Annals of Allergy, Asthma, and Immunology,* 1999; 82:185–91.

Gordon, A., et al. "Creatine Supplementation in Chronic Heart Failure Increases Skeletal Muscle Creatine Phosphate and Muscle Performance." *Cardiovascular Research,* 1995; 30:413–18.

Hagen, T. M., J. Liu, J. Lukkesfeldt, et al. "Feeding Acetyl-L-Carnitine and Lipoic Acid to Old Rats Significantly Improves Metabolic Function While Decreasing Oxidative Stress." *Proceedings of the National Academy of Sciences of the USA,* 2002; 99:1870–75.

Langsjoen, P. H., and Langsjoen, A. M. "The Clinical Use of HMG CoA-Reductase Inhibitors and the Associated Depletion of Coenzyme Q10. A Review of Animal and Human Publications." *BioFactors,* 2003; 18:101–11.

Lockwood, K., S. Moesgaard, T. Yamamoto, et al. "Progress on Therapy of Breast Cancer with Vitamin Q10 and the Regression of Metastases." *Biochemical and Biophysical Research Communications,* 1995; 212:172–77.

Mizuno, M., B. Quistorff, H. Theorell, et al. "Effects of Oral Supplementation of Coenzyme Q10 on 31P-NMR Detected Skeletal Muscle Energy Metabolism In Middle-Aged Post-Polio Subjects and Normal Volunteers." *Molecular Aspects of Medicine,* 1997; 18 (Suppl):S291–98.

Musumeci, O., A. Naini, A. E. Slonin, et al. "Familial Cerebellar Ataxia with Muscle Coenzyme Q10 Deficiency." *Neurology,* 2001; 56:849–55.

Plioplys, A. V., and S. Plioplys. "Amantadine and L-Carnitine Treatment of Chronic Fatigue Syndrome." *Neuropsychobiology,* 1997; 35:16–23.

Shults, C. W., D. Oakes, K. Kieburtz, et al. "Effects of Coenzyme Q10 in Early Parkinson Disease. Evidence of Slowing of the Functional Decline." *Archives of Neurology,* 2002; 59;1541–50.

Kuratsune, H., et al. "Acylcarnitine Deficiency in Chronic Fatigue Syndrome." *Clinical Infectious Diseases,* 1994; 18 (Suppl 1)S62–67.

Liu, J., E. Head, A. M. Gharib, et al. "Memory Loss in Old Rats Is Associated with Brain Mitochondrial Decay and RNA/DNA Oxidation: Partial Reversal by Feeding Acetyl-L-Carnitine and/or R-A-Lipoic Acid." *Proceedings of the National Academy of Sciences*, 2002; 99:2356–61.

————, D. W. Killilea, and B. N. Ames. "Age-Associated Mitochondrial Oxidative Decay: Improvement of Carnitine Acetyltransferase Substrate-Binding Affinity and Activity in Brain by Feeding Old Rats Acetyl-L-Carnitine and/or R-A-Lipoic Acid." *Proceedings of the National Academy of Sciences of the USA*, 2002; 99:1876–81.

Omran, H., S. Illien, D. MacCarter, et al. "D-Ribose Improves Diastolic Function and Quality of Life in Congestive Heart Failure Patients: A Prospective Feasibility Study." *European Journal of Heart Failure*, 2003; 5:615–19.

Stockler, S., et al. "Creatine Replacement Therapy in Guanidinoacetate Methyltransferase Deficiency, A Novel Inborn Error of Metabolism." *Lancet*, 1996; 348:789–90.

Thal, L. J., A. Carta, W. R. Clarke, et al. "A 1-Year Multicenter Placebo-Controlled Study of Acetyl-L-Carnitine in Patients with Alzheimer's Disease." *Neurology*, 1996; 47:705–11.

Van Gammerren, D., D. Falk, and J. Antonio. "The Effects of Four Weeks of Ribose Supplementation on Body Composition and Exercise Performance in Healthy, Young, Male Recreational Bodybuilders: A Double-Blind, Placebo-Controlled Trial." *Current Therapeutic Research—Clinical and Experimental*, 2002; 63:486–95.

Volek, J. S., et al. "Creatine Supplementation Enhances Muscular Performance during High-Intensity Resistance Exercise." *Journal of the American Dietetic Association*, July 1997; 97:765–70.

CHAPTER 5. NUTRIENTS THAT MAKE AND REPAIR DNA

Ames, B. N. "Cancer Prevention and Diet: Help from Single Nucleotide Polymorphisms." *Proceedings of the National Academy of Sciences*, 1999; 96:12216–18.

Blount, B. C., M. M. Mack, C. M. Wehr, et al. "Folate Deficiency Causes Uracil Misincorporation into Human DNA and Chromosome Breakage: Implications for Cancer and Neuronal Damage." *Proceedings of the National Academy of Sciences*, 1997; 94:3290–95.

Collins, A. R., V. Harrington, J. Drew, et al. "Nutritional Modulation of DNA Repair in a Human Intervention Study." *Carcinogenesis*, 2003; 24:511–15.

Cooney, C. A., A. A. Dave, and G. L. Wolff. "Maternal Methyl Supplements in Mice Affect Epigenetic Variation and DNA Methylation of Offspring." *Journal of Nutrition*, 2002; 132:2392S–2400S.

Fenech, M., C. Aitken, and J. Rinaldi. "Folate, Vitamin B12, Homocysteine Status and DNA Damage in Young Australian Adults." *Carcinogenesis*, 1998; 19:1163–71.

Jacobson, E. L., A. J. Dame, J. S. Pyrek, et al. "Evaluating the Role of Niacin in Human Carcinogenesis." *Biochemie*, 1995; 77:394–98.

Johanning, G. L., D. C. Heimburger, and C. J. Piyathilake. "DNA Methylation and Diet in Cancer." *Journal of Nutrition*, 2002; 132:3814S–18S.

Kimura, M., K. Umegaki, M. Higuchi, et al. "Methylenetetrahydrofolate Reductase C677T Polymorphism, Folic Acid and Riboflavin Are Important Determinants of Genome Stability in Cultured Human Lymphocytes." *Journal of Nutrition*, 2004; 134:48–56.

Schnyder, G., M. Roffi, Y. Flammer, et al. "Effect of Homocysteine-Lowering Therapy with Folic Acid, Vitamin B_{12}, and Vitamn B_6 on Clinical Outcome after Percutaneous Coronary Intervention. The Swiss Heart Study: A Randomized Controlled Trial." *Journal of the American Medical Association*, 2002; 288:973–79.

Spronck, J. C., A. P. Batleman, A. C. Boyonoski, et al. "Chronic DNA Damage and Niacin Deficiency Enhance Cell Injury and Cause Unusual Interactions in NAD and Poly(ADP-Ribose) Metabolism in Rat Bone Marrow." *Nutrition and Cancer*, 2003; 45:124–31.

Webster, R. P., M. D. Gawde, and R. K. Bhattacharya. "Modulation of Carcinogen-Induced DNA Damage and Repair Enzyme Activity by Dietary Riboflavin." *Cancer Letters*, 1996; 98:129–35.

Wald, D. S., M. Law, and J. K. Morris. "Homocysteine and Cardiovascular Disease: Evidence on Causality from a Meta-Analysis." *British Medical Journal*, 2002; 325:1202–8.

Waterland, R. A., and R. L. Jirtle. "Transposable Elements: Targets for Early Nutritional Effects on Epigenetic Gene Regulation." *Molecular and Cellular Biology*, 2003; 23:5293–5300.

CHAPTER 6. NUTRIENTS THAT PROTECT DNA FROM DAMAGE

Archer, S. Y., S. Meng, A. Shei, et al. "p21 WAFI Is Required for Butyrate-Mediated Growth Inhibition of Human Colon Cancer Cells." *Proceedings of the National Academy of Sciences of the USA*, 1998; 95:6791–96.

Beck, M. A., Q. Shi, V. C. Morris, et al. "Rapid Genomic Evolution of a Non-Virulent Coxsackievirus B3 in Selenium-Deficient Mice Results in Selection of Identical Virulent Isolates." *Nature Medicine*, May 1995; 1:433–36.

Bertram, J. S. "Carotenoids and Gene Regulation." *Nutrition Reviews*, 1999; 57:182–91.

Challem, J. J., and E. W. Taylor. "Retroviruses, Ascorbate, and Mutations, in the Evolution of Homo Sapiens." *Free Radical Biology and Medicine*, 1998; 25:130–32.

Clark, L. C., G. F. Combs Jr, B. W. Turnbull, et al. "Effects of Selenium Supplementation for Cancer Prevention in Patients with Carcinoma of the Skin. A Randomized Controlled Trial." Nutritional Prevention of Cancer Study Group. *Journal of the American Medical Association*, 1996; 276:1957–63.

De Flora, S., C. F. Cesarone, R. Balanksy, et al. "Chemopreventive Properties and Mechanisms of N-Acetylcysteine. The Experimental Background." *Journal of Cellular Biochemistry*, 1995; Suppl 22:33–41.

———, C. Grassi, and L. Carati. "Attenuation of Influenza-like Symptomatology and Improvement of Cell-Mediated Immunity with Long-Term N-Acetylcysteine Treatment." *European Respiratory Journal*, 1997; 10:1535–41.

Devaraj, S., and I. Jialal. "Alpha Tocopherol Supplementation Decreases Serum C-Reactive Protein and Monocyte Interleukin-6 Levels in Normal Volunteers and Type 2 Diabetic Patients." *Free Radical Biology and Medicine*, 2000; 29:790–92.

Duffy, S. J., N. Gokce, M. Holbrook, et al. "Treatment of Hypertension with Ascorbic Acid." *Lancet*, 1999; 354:2048–49.

Dusinska, M., A. Kazimirova, M. Barancokova, et al. "Nutritional Supplementation with Antioxidants Decreases Chromosomal Damage in Humans." *Mutagenesis*, 2003; 18:371–76.

Edmonds, S. E., P. G. Yinyard, R. Guo, et al. "Putative Analgesic Activity of Repeated Oral Doses of Vitamin E in the Treatment of Rheumatoid Arthritis. Results of a Prospective Placebo-Controlled Double-Blind Trial." *Annals of the Rheumatic Diseases*, 1997; 56:649–55.

Emerit, I., N. Oganesian, T. Sarkisian, et al. "Clastogenic Factors in the Plasma of Chernobyl Accident Recovery Workers: Anticlastogenic Effect of Ginkgo Biloba Extract." *Radiation Research*, 1995; 144:198–205.

Engelhart, M. J., M. I. Geerlings, A. Ruitenberg, et al. "Dietary Intake of Antioxidants and Risk of Alzheimer's Disease." *Journal of the American Medical Association*, 2002; 287:3223–29.

Frydoonfar, H. R., D. R. McGrath, and A. D. Spigelman. "The Variable Effect on Proliferation of a Colon Cancer Cell Line by the Citrus Fruit Flavonoid Naringenin." *Colorectal Diseases*, 2003; 5:149–52.

Fuller, C. J., B. A. Huet, and I. Jialal. "Effects of Increasing Doses of Alpha-Tocopherol in Providing Protection of Low-Density Lipoprotein from Oxidation." *American Journal of Cardiology*, 1998; 81:231–33.

Giovannucci, E. "Tomatoes, Tomato-Based Products, Lycopene, and Cancer: Review of the Epidemiologic Literature." *Journal of the National Cancer Institute*, 1999; 91:317–31.

Haney, D. Q. "Tomato Nutrient May Fight Cancer." Associated Press, April 13, 1999.

Helmy, M., M. Shohayeb, M. H. Helmy, et al. "Antioxidants as Adjuvant Therapy in Rheumatoid Disease—a Preliminary Study." *Arzneimittel-Forschung/Drug Research*, 2001; 51:293–98.

Hemilä, H. "Does Vitamin C Alleviate the Symptoms of the Common Cold? A Review of Current Evidence." *Scandinavian Journal of Infectious Diseases*, January 1994; 26:1–6.

Herzenberg, L. A., S. C. De Rosa, J. G. Dubs, et al. "Glutathione Deficiency Is Associated with Impaired Survival in HIV Disease." *Proceedings of the National Academy of Sciences of the USA*, 1997; 94:1967–72.

Jackson, M. J., A. McArdle, and F. McArdle. "Antioxidant Micronutrients and Gene Expression." *Proceedings of the Nutrition Society*, 1998; 57:301–5.

Khaw, K. T., S. Bingham, A. Welch, et al. "Relation between Plasma Ascorbic Acid and Mortality in Men and Women in EPIC-Norfolk Prospective Study: A Prospective Population Study." *Lancet*, 2001; 357:657–63.

Kucuk, O., F. H. Sarkar, et al. "Effects of Lycopene Supplementation in Patients with Localized Prostate Cancer." *Experimental Biology and Medicine*, 2002; 227(10): 881–85.

Morris, M. C., D. A. Evans, J. L. Bienias, et al. "Vitamin E and Cognitive Decline in Older Persons." *Archives of Neurology*, 2002; 59:1125–32.

Nelson, H. K., Q. Shi, P. Van Dael, et al. "Host Nutritional Selenium Status As a Driving Force for Influenza Virus Mutations." *FASEB Journal*, 2001; 15:1481–83.

Ortega, R. M., A. M. Requejo, A. M. Lopez-Sobaler, et al. "Cognitive Function in Elderly People Is Influenced by Vitamin E Status." *Journal of Nutrition*, 2002; 132:2065–68.

Padayatty, S. J., and M. Levine. "New Insights into the Physiology and Pharmacology of Vitamin C." *Canadian Medical Association Journal*, 2001; 164:353–55.

Palmer, H. J., and K. E. Paulson. "Reactive Oxygen Species and Antioxidants in Signal Transduction and Gene Expression." *Nutrition Reviews*, 1997; 55:353–61.

Rihn, B., C. Saliou, M. C. Bottin, et al. "From Ancient Remedies to Modern Therapeutics: Pine Bark Uses in Skin Disorders Revisited." *Phytotherapy Research*, 2001; 15:76–78.

Rudolph, R. E., T. L. Vaughan, A. R. Kristal, et al. "Serum Selenium Levels in Relation to Markers of Neoplastic Progression among Persons with Barrett's Esophagus." *Journal of the National Cancer Institute*, 2003; 95:750–57.

Sano, M., C. Ernesto, R. G. Thomas, et al. "A Controlled Trial of Selegiline, Alpha-tocopherol, or Both as Treatment for Alzheimer's Disease." *New England Journal of Medicine*, 1997; 336:1216–22.

Stivala, L. A., M. Savio, A. Quarta, et al. "The Antiproliferative Effect of b-Carotene Requires p21 waf1/cip1 in Normal Human Fibroblasts." *European Journal of Biochemistry*, 2000; 267:2290–96.

Sweetman, S. F., J. J. Strain, and V. J. McKelvey-Martin. "Effect of Antioxidant Vitamin Supplementation on DNA Damage and Repair in Human Lymphoblastoid Cells." *Nutrition and Cancer*, 1997; 27:122–30.

Takahashi, T., C. Schulze, B. Lord, et al. "Ascorbic Acid Enhances Differentiation of Embryonic Stem Cells into Cardiac Myocytes." *Circulation*, March 31, 2003: electronic publication in advance of print.

Upritchard, J. E., W. H. F. Sutherland, and J. I. Mann. "Effect of Supplementation with Tomato Juice, Vitamin E, and Vitamin C on LDL Oxidation and Products of Inflammatory Activity in Type 2 Diabetes." *Diabetes Care*, 2000; 23:733–38.

Virgili, F., H. Kobuchi, and L. Packer. "Procyanidins Extracted from Pinus Maritima (Pycnogenol [R]): Scavengers of Free Radical Species and Modulators of Nitrogen Monoxide Metabolism in Activated Murine Raw 264.7 Macrophages." *Free Radical Biology and Medicine*, 1998; 24:1120–29.

Watanabe, C. M. H., S. Wolffram, P. Ader, et al. "The In Vivo Neuromodulatory Effects of the Herbal Medicine Ginkgo Biloba." *Proceedings of the National Academy of Sciences*, 2001; 98:6577–80.

Zandi, P. P., H. J. C. Anthony, A. S. Khachaturian, et al. "Reduced Risk of Alzheimer Disease in Users of Antioxidant Vitamin Supplements. The Cache County Study." *Archives of Neurology*, 2004; 61:82–88.

Zi, X., D. K. Feyes, and R. Agarwal. "Anticarcinogenic Effect of a Flavonoid Antioxidant, Silymarin, in Human Breast Cancer Cells MDA-MB 468." *Cancer Research*, 1998; 58: 1920–29.

CHAPTER 7. DIETARY GUIDELINES FOR FEEDING YOUR GENES RIGHT

Asami, D. K., Y. J. Hong, D. M. Barrett, et al. "Comparison of the Total Phenolic and Ascorbic Acid Content of Freeze-Dried and Air-Dried Marionberry, Strawberry, and Corn Grown Using Conventional, Organic, and Sustainable Agriculture Practices." *Journal of Agricultural and Food Chemistry*, 2003; 51:1237–41.

Goldman, R., and P. G. Shields. "Food Mutagens." *Journal of Nutrition*, 2003; 133(Suppl):965S–73S.

Hays, J. H., A. DiSabatino, R. T. Gorman, et al. "Effect of a High Saturated Fat and No-Starch Diet on Serum Lipid Subfractions in Patients with Documented Atherosclerotic Cardiovascular Disease." *Mayo Clinic Proceedings*, 2003; 78;1331–36.

Hu, F. B., L. Bronner, W. C. Willett, et al. "Fish and Omega-3 Fatty Acid Intake and Risk of Coronary Heart Disease in Women. *Journal of the American Medical Association*, 2002; 287:1815–21.

Nestel, P., H. Shige, S. Pomeroy, et al. "The n-3 Fatty Acids Eicosapentaenoic Acid and Docosahexaenoic Acid Increase System Arterial Compliance in Humans." *American Journal of Clinical Nutrition*, 2002; 76:326–30.

Uribarri, J., M. Peppa, W. Cai, et al. "Restriction of Dietary Glycotoxins Reduces Excessive Advanced Glycation End Products in Renal Failure Patients." *Journal of the American Society of Nephrology*, 2003; 14:728–31.

CHAPTER 9. STRESS, GENES, AND NUTRITION

Benton, D., J. Haller, and J. Fordy. "Vitamin Supplementation for 1 Year Improves Mood." *Neuropsychobiology*, 1995; 32:98–105.

Benton, D., R. Griffiths, and J. Haller. "Thiamine Supplementation Mood and Cognitive Functioning." *Psychopharmacology*, 1997; 129:66–71.

Bjelland, I., G. S. Tell, S. E. Vollset, et al. "Folate, Vitamin B12, Homocysteine, and the MTHFR 677C–T Polymorphism in Anxiety and Depression." *Archives of General Psychiatry*, 2003; 60:618–26.

Black, P. H., and L. D. Garbutt. "Stress, Inflammation and Cardiovascular Disease." *Journal of Psychosomatic Research*, 2002; 52:1–23.

Bower, B. "Worried to Death: Lifelong Inhibitions Hasten Rodents' Deaths." *Science News*, 2003; 164:373.

Brody, S. "High-Dose Ascorbic Acid Increases Intercourse Frequency and Improves Mood: A Randomized Controlled Clinical Trial." *Biological Psychiatry*, 2002; 52:371–74.

Caspi, A., K. Sugden, T. E. Moffitt, et al. "Influence of Life Stress on Depression: Moderation by a Polymorphism in the 5-HTT Gene." *Science*, 2003; 301:386–89.

Elmadfa, I., D. Jajchrzak, P. Rust, et al. "The Thiamine Status of Adult Humans Depends on Carbohydrate Intake." *International Journal for Vitamin and Nutrition Research*, 2001; 71:217–21.

Kakuda, T., A. Nozawa, T. Unno, et al. "Inhibiting Effects of Theanine on Caffeine Stimulation Evaluated by EEG in the Rat." *Biosci Biotechnol Biochem*, 2000; 64:287–93.

Kiecolt–Glaser, J. K., K. J. Preacher, R. C. MacCallum, et al. "Chronic Stress and Age-Related Increases in the Proinflammatory Cytokines IL-6." *Proceedings of the National Academy of Sciences*, 2003: epub ahead of print.

Leventhal, A. G., Y. Wang, M. Pu, et al. "GABA and Its Antagonists Improved Visual Cortical Function in Senescent Monkeys." *Science*, 2003; 300:812–15.

Palatnik, A., K. Prolov, M. Fux, et al. "Double-Blind, Controlled Crossover Trial of Inositol versus Fluvoxamine for the Treatment of Panic Disorder." *Journal of Clinical Psychopharmacology*, 2001; 21:335–39.

Rossi E. *The Psychobiology of Gene Expression: Neuroscience and Neurogenesis in Hypnosis and the Healing Arts.* New York: W. W. Norton Professional Books, 2002.

Salzano, J. "Taming Stress." *Scientific American*, September 2003: 87–95.

Santarelli, L., M. Saxe, C. Gross, et al. "Requirement of Hippocampal Neurogenesis for the Behavioral Effects of Antidepressants." *Science*, 2003; 301:805–9.

Yokogoshi, H., Y. Kato, Y. M. Sagesaka, et al. "Reduction Effect of Theanine on Blood Pressure and Brain 5-Hydroxyindoles in Spontaneously Hypertensive Rats." *Biosci Biotechnol Biochem*, 1995; 59:615–18.

Williams, R. B., J. C. Carefoot, and N. Schneiderman. "Psychological Risk Factors for Cardiovascular Disease. More Than One Culprit at Work." *Journal of the American Medical Association*, 2003; 290:2190–92.

CHAPTER 10. NUTRITIONAL RECOMMENDATIONS FOR SPECIFIC DISEASES, A TO Z

Temple, L. K., R. S. McLeod, S. Gallinger, et al. "Defining Disease in the Genomics Era." *Science*, 2001; 293:807–8.

AGING

Ames, B. N. "Micronutrients Prevent Cancer and Delay Aging." *Toxicology Letters*, 1998; 102–103:5–18.

Harman, D. "Free Radical Theory of Aging." *Mutation Research*, 1992; 275:257–66.

———. "Aging: Phenomena and Theories." *Annals of the New York Academy of Sciences*, 1998; 854:1–7.

Purba, M., A. Kouris-Blazos, N. Wattanapenpaiboon, et al. "Skin Wrinkling: Can Food Make a Difference?" *Journal of the American College of Nutrition*, 2001; 20:71–80.

ALZHEIMER'S DISEASE

Clark, R., A. D. Smith, K. A. Jobst, et al. "Folate, Vitamin B_{12}, and Serum Total Homocysteine Levels in Confirmed Alzheimer's Disease." *Archives of Neurology*, 1998; 55:1449–55.

Engelhart, M. J., M. I. Geerlings, A. Ruitenberg, et al. "Dietary Intake of Antioxidants and Risk of Alzheimer's Disease." *Journal of the American Medical Association*, 2002; 287:3223–29.

Hager, K., A. Marahrens, M. Kenklies, et al. "Alpha-Lipoic Acid as a New Treatment Option for Alzheimer Type Dementia." *Archives of Gerontology and Geriatrics*, 2001; 32:275–82.

LeBars, P. L., M. M. Katz, N. Berman, et al. "A Placebo-Controlled, Double-Blind Randomized Trial of an Extract of *Ginkgo Biloba* for Dementia." *Journal of the American Medical Association*, 1997; 278:1327–32.

Liu, J., E. Head, A. M. Gharib, et al. "Memory Loss in Old Rats Is Associated with Brain Mitochondrial Decay and RNA/DNA Oxidation: Partial Reversal by Feeding Acetyl-L-Carnitine and/or R-A-Lipoic Acid." *Proceedings of the National Academy of Sciences*, 2002; 99:2356–61.

Morris, M. C., D. A. Evans, J. L. Bienias, et al. "Dietary Intake of Antioxidant Nutrients and the Risk of Incident Alzheimer's Disease in a Biracial Community Study." *Journal of the American Medical Association*, 2002; 287:3230–37.

Sano, M., C. Ernesto, R. G. Thomas, et al. "A Controlled Trial of Selegiline, Alpha-Tocopherol, or Both as Treatment for Alzheimer's Disease." *New England Journal of Medicine*, 1997; 336:1216–22.

Selhub, J., L. C. Bagley, J. Miller, et al. "B Vitamins, Homocysteine, and Neurocognitive Function in the Elderly." *American Journal of Clinical Nutrition*, 2000; 71(suppl): 614S–20S.

Seshadri, S., A. Beiser, J. Selhub, et al. "Plasma Homocysteine as a Risk Factor for Dementia and Alzheimer's Disease." *New England Journal of Medicine*, 2002; 346:476–83.

Zandi, P. P., H. J. C. Anthony, A. S. Khachaturian, et al. "Reduced Risk of Alzheimer Disease in Users of Antioxidant Vitamin Supplements. The Cache County Study." *Archives of Neurology*, 2004; 61:82–88.

BIRTH DEFECTS

Bennett, M. "Vitamin B12 Deficiency, Infertility and Recurrent Fetal Loss." *Journal of Reproductive Medicine*, 2001; 46:209–12.

Busciglio, J., and B. A. Yankner. "Apoptosis and Increased Generation of Reactive Oxygen Species in Down's Syndrome Neurons In Vitro." *Nature*, 1995; 378: 776–79.

Loffredo, L. C. M., J. M. P. Souza, J. A. S. Freitas, et al. "Oral Clefts and Vitamin Supplementation." *Cleft Palate—Cranialfacial Journal*, 2001; 38:76–83.

MacLeod, K. *Down Syndrome and Vitamin Therapy*. Canada: Kemanso Publishing, 2003.

Preston-Martin, S., J. M. Pogoda, B. A. Mueller, et al. "Prenatal Vitamin Supplementation and Risk of Childhood Brain Tumors." *International Journal of Cancer*, 1998; 11:17–22.

Turkel, H., and I. Nusbaum. *Medical Treatment of Down Syndrome and Genetic Diseases*. Southfield, MI: Ubiotica, 1985.

van Rooij, I. A. L. M., C. Vermeij-Keers, L. A. J. Kluijtmans, et al. "Does the Interaction between Maternal Folate Intake and the Methylenetetrahydrofolate Reductase Polymnorphisms Affect the Risk of Cleft Lip with or without Cleft Palate?" *American Journal of Epidemiology*, 2003; 157:583–91.

Shaw, G. M., T. Quach, V. Nelson, et al. "Neural Tube Defects Associated with Maternal Periconceptional Dietary Intake of Simple Sugars and Glycemic Index." *American Journal of Clinical Nutrition*, 2003; 78:972–78.

CANCER

Boileau, T. W. M., Z. Liao, S. Kim, et al. "Prostate Carcinogenesis in N-methyl-N-nitrosourea (NMU)—Testosterone-Treated Rats Fed Tomato Powder, Lycopene, or Energy-Restricted Diets." *Journal of the National Cancer Institute*, 2003; 95:1578–86.

Clark, L. C., G. F. Combs Jr, B. W. Turnbull, et al. "Effects of Selenium Supplementation for Cancer Prevention in Patients with Carcinoma of the Skin. A Randomized Controlled Trial." Nutritional Prevention of Cancer Study Group. *Journal of the American Medical Association*, 1996; 276:1957–63.

Drisko, J. A., J. Chapman, V. J. Hunter. "The Use of Antioxidants with First-Line Chemotherapy in Two Cases of Ovarian Cancer." *Journal of the American College of Nutrition*, 2003; 22:118–23.

Giovannucci, E., A. Ascherio, E. B. Rimm, et al. "Intake of Carotenoids and Retinol in Relation to Risk of Prostate Cancer." *Journal of the National Cancer Institute*, 1995; 87:1767–76.

Hartman, T. J., D. Albanes, P. Pietinen, et al. "The Association between Baseline Vitamin E, Selenium, and Prostate Cancer in the Alpha-Tocopherol, Beta-Carotene Cancer Prevention Study." *Cancer Epidemiology, Biomarkers and Prevention*, 1998; 7:335–40.

Kim, Y. I. "Methylenetetrahydrofolate Reductase Polymorphisms, Folate, and Cancer Risk: A Paradigm of Gene-Nutrient Interactions in Carcinogenesis." *Nutrition Reviews*, 2000; 58:205–17.

———, I. P. Pogribny, A. G. Basnakian, et al. "Folate Deficiency in Rats Induces DNA Strand Breaks and Hypomethylation within the p53 Tumor Suppressor Genes." *American Journal of Clinical Nutrition*, 1997; 65:46–52.

Kucuk, O., F. H. Sarker, Z. Djuric, et al. "Effects of Lycopene Supplementation in Patients with Localized Prostate Cancer." *Experimental Biology and Medicine*, 2002; 227:881–85.

Lockwood, K., S. Moesgaard, and K. Folkers. "Partial and Complete Regression of Breast Cancer in Patients in Relation to Dosage of Coenzyme Q10." *Biochemical and Biophysical Research Communications*, 1994; 199:1504–8.

Patterson, R. E., E. White, A. R. Kristal, et al. "Vitamin Supplements and Cancer Risk: The Epidemiological Evidence." *Cancer Causes and Control*, 1997; 8:786–802.

Prasad, K. N., B. Kumar, X. D. Yan, et al. "a-Tocopherol Succinate, the Most Effective Form of Vitamin E for Adjuvant Cancer Treatment: A Review." *Journal of the American College of Nutrition*, 2003; 22:108–17.

CARDIOVASCULAR DISEASES

Boaz, M., S. Smetana, T. Weinstein, et al. "Secondary Prevention with Antioxidants of Cardiovascular Disease in Endstage Renal Disease (SPACE): Randomised Placebo-Controlled Trial." *Lancet*, 2000; 356:1213–18.

Boushey, C. J., et al. "A Quantitative Assessment of Plasma Homocysteine as a Risk Factor for Vascular Disease." *Journal of the American Medical Association*, 1995; 274:1049–57.

Buffon, A., L. M. Biasucci, G. Liuzzo, et al. "Widespread Coronary Inflammation in Unstable Angina." *New England Journal of Medicine*, 2002; 347:5–12.

Duffy, S. J., N. Gokce, M. Holbrook, et al. "Treatment of Hypertension with Ascorbic Acid." *Lancet*, 1999; 354:2048–49.

Hays, J. H., A. DiSabatino, R. T. Gorman, et al. "Effect of a High Saturated Fat and No-Starch Diet on Serum Lipid Subfractions in Patients with Documented Atherosclerotic Cardiovascular Disease." *Mayo Clinic Proceedings*, 2003; 78;1331–36.

Hu, F. B., L. Bronner, W. C. Willett, et al. "Fish and Omega-3 Fatty Acid Intake and Risk of Coronary Heart Disease in Women." *Journal of the American Medical Association*, 2002; 287:1815–21.

Jialal, I., M. Traber, and S. Deveraj. "Is There a Vitamin E Paradox?" *Current Opinion in Lipidology*, 2001; 12:49–53.

Kurl, S., T. P. Tuomainen, J. A. Laukkanen, et al. "Plasma Vitamin C Modifies the Association between Hypertension and Risk of Stroke." *Stroke*, 2002; 33:1568–73.

Lobo, A., A. Naso, and K. Aheart. "Reduction of Homocysteine Levels in Coronary Artery Disease by Low-Dose Folic Acid Combined with Vitamin B_6 and B_{12}." *American Journal of Cardiology*, 1999; 83:821–25.

Loria, C. M., D. D. Ingram, J. J. Feldman, et al. "Serum Folate and Cardiovascular Disease Mortality among U.S. Men and Women." *Archives of Internal Medicine*, 2000; 160;3258–62.

McCully, K. S. "Homocysteinemia and Arteriosclerosis." *American Heart Journal*, 1972; 83:571–73.

———. "Homocystine, Atherosclerosis and Thrombosis: Implications for Oral Contraceptive Users." *American Journal of Clinical Nutrition*, 1975; 28:542–49.

———. "Vascular Pathology of Homocysteinemia: Implications for the Pathogenesis of Arteriosclerosis." *American Journal of Pathology*, 1969; 56:111–28.

Morris, M. C., D. A. Evans, J. L. Bienias, et al. "Dietary Intake of Antioxidant Nutrients and the Risk of Incident Alzheimer's Disease in a Biracial Community Study." *Journal of the American Medical Association*, 2002; 287:3230–37.

———. "Vitamin E and Cognitive Decline in Older Persons." *Archives of Neurology*, 2002; 59:1125–32.

Nestel, P., H. Shige, S. Pomeroy, et al. "The n-3 Fatty Acids Eicosapentaenoic Acid and Docosahexaenoic Acid Increase System Arterial Compliance in Humans." *American Journal of Clinical Nutrition*, 2002; 76:326–30.

Plotnick, G. D., M. C. Corretti, and R. A. Vogel. "Effect of Antioxidant Vitamins on the Transient Impairment of Endothelium-Dependent Brachial Artery Vasoactivity following a Single High-Fat Meal." *Journal of the American Medical Association*, 1997; 278:1682–86.

Ridker, P. M., C. H. Hennekens, J. E. Buring, et al. "C-Reactive Protein and Other Markers of Inflammation in the Prediction of Cardiovascular Disease in Women." *New England Journal of Medicine*, 2000; 342:836–43.

Salonen, J. T., K. Nyyssonen, R. Salonen, et al. "Antioxidant Supplementation in Atherosclerosis Prevention (ASAP) Study: A Randomized Trial of the Effect of Vitamins E and C on 3-Year Progression of Carotid Atherosclerosis." *Journal of Internal Medicine*, 2000; 248:377–86.

Stephens, N. G., A. Parsons, P. M. Schofield, et al. "Randomized Controlled Trial of Vitamin E in Patients with Coronary Disease: Cambridge Heart Antioxidant Study (CHAOS)." *Lancet*, 1996; 347:781–86.

Wald, D. S., M. Law, and J. K. Morris. "Homocysteine and Cardiovascular Disease: Evidence on Causality from a Meta-Analysis." *British Medical Journal*, 2002; 325:1202–8.

Warsi, A. A., B. Davies, and G. Morris-Stiff. "Abdominal Aortic Aneurysm and Its Correlation to Plasma Homocysteine and Vitamins." *European Journal of Vascular and Endovascular Surgery*, 2004; 27:75–79.

CARDIOMYOPATHY AND HEART FAILURE

Bliznakov, E. G., and D. J. Wilkins. "Biochemical and Clinical Consequences of Inhibiting Coenzyme Q10 Biosynthesis by Lipid-Lowering HMG-CoA Reductase Inhibitors (Statins): A Critical Overview." *Advances in Therapy*, 1998; 15:218–28.

Folkers, K., P. Langsjoen, and P. H. Langsjoen. "Therapy with Coenzyme Q10 of Patients in Heart Failure Who Are Eligible or Ineligible for a Transplant." *Biochemical and Biophysical Research Communications*, 1992; 182:247–53.

Fosslien, E. "Mitochondrial Medicine—Cardiomyopathy Caused by Defective Oxida-

SELECTED REFERENCES 237

tive Phosphorylation." *Annals of Clinical and Laboratory Science,* 2003; 33: 371–95.
Langsjoen, P. H., A. Langsjoen, R. Willis, et al. "Treatment of Hypertrophic Cardiomy-
opathy with Coenzyme Q10." *Molecular Aspects of Medicine,* 1997;18 (Suppl):
S145–51.
Leslie, D., and M. Gheorghiade. "Is There a Role for Thiamine Supplementation in the
Management of Heart Failure." *American Heart Journal,* 19996; 131:1248–50.
Rizos, I. "Three-Year Survival of Patients with Heart Failure Caused by Dilated Car-
diomyopathy and L-Carnitine Administration." *American Heart Journal,* 2000;
139:S120–23.
Sarter, B. "Coenzyme Q10 and Cardiovascular Disease: A Review." *Journal of Cardio-
vascular Nursing,* 2002; 16: 9–20.

CELIAC DISEASE

Banco, G. "Conditions and Disorders Associated with Celiac Disease." *Journal of Pedi-
atric Gastroenterology and Nutrition,* 2000; 31(Suppl 3):S28, Abstract #100.
Braly, J., and R. Hoggan. *Dangerous Grains.* New York: Penguin Putnam, 2002.
Cicarelli, G., G. Della Rocca, M. Amboni, et al. "Clinical and Neurological Abnormali-
ties in Adult Celiac Disease." *Neurological Sciences,* 2003; 24:311–17.
Cordain, L., J. B. Miller, S. B. Eaton, et al. "Plant-Animal Subsistence Ratios and
Macronutrient Energy Estimates in Worldwide Hunter-Gatherer Diets." *American
Journal of Clinical Nutrition,* 2000; 71:682–92.
Eaton, S. B., and S. B. Eaton II. "Paleolithic vs. Modern Diets—Selected Pathophysical
Implications." *European Journal of Nutrition,* 2000; 39:67–70.
Fasano, A. "Celiac Disease—How to Handle a Clinical Chameleon." *New England
Journal of Medicine,* 2003; 348:2568–70.
Hadjivassiliou, M., R. A. Grunewald, and G. A. Davies-Jones. "Gluten Sensitivity: A
Many-Headed Hydra." *British Medical Journal,* 1999; 318:1710–11.
McManus, R., and D. Kelleher. "Celiac Disease—the Villain Unmasked?" *New
England Journal of Medicine,* 2003; 348:2573–74.
Smith, M. D. *Going Against the Grain.* Chicago: Contemporary Books, 2002.

DEPRESSION AND MOODINESS

Benton, D., R. Griffiths, and J. Haller. "Thiamine Supplementation, Mood and Cognitive Functioning." *Psychopharmacology,* 1997; 129:66–71.
———, J. Haller, and J. Fordy. "Vitamin Supplementation for 1 Year Improves Mood."
Neuropsychobiology, 1995; 32:98–105.
Brenner, R., V. Azbel, S. Madhusoodanan, et al. "Comparison of an Extract of Hyper-
icum (LI 160) and Sertraline in the Treatment of Depression: A Double-Blind, Ran-
domized Pilot Study." *Clinical Therapeutics,* 2000; 22:411–19.
Caspi, A., K. Sugden, T. E. Moffitt, et al. "Influence of Life Stress on Depression: Mod-
eration by a Polymorphism in the 5-HTT Gene." *Science,* 2003; 301:386–89.
Schrader, E. "Equivalence of St. John's Wort Extract (Ze 117) and Fluoxetine: A
Randomized Controlled Study in Mild-Moderate Depression." *International Clinical Psychopharmacology,* 2000; 15:61–68.

FATIGUE AND CHRONIC FATIGUE

Barbiroli, B., R. Medori, H. J. Tritschler, et al. "Lipoic (Thioctic) Acid Increases Brain
Energy Availability and Skeletal Muscle Performance as Shown by In Vivo 31P-MRS
in a Patient with Mitochondrial Cytopathy." *Journal of Neurology,* 1995; 242:472–77.
Heap, L. C., T. J. Peters, S. Wessely. "Vitamin B Status in Patients with Chronic Fatigue
Syndrome." *Journal of the Royal Society of Medicine,* 1999; 92:183–85.

Plioplys, A. V., and S. Plioplys. "Amantadine and L-Carnitine Treatment of Chronic Fatigue Syndrome. *Neuropsychobiology*, 1997; 35:16–23.

Sinatra, S. T. "Coenzyme Q10: A Vital Therapeutic Nutrient for the Heart with Special Application in Congestive Heart Failure." *Connecticut Medicine*, 1997; 61:707–11.

HEMOCHROMATOSIS

Heath, A. L. M., and S. J. Fairweather. "Health Implications of Iron Overload: The Role of Diet and Genotype." *Nutrition Reviews*, 2003; 61:45–62.

Kaltwasser, J. P., E. Werner, K. Schalk, et al. "Clinical Trial on the Effect of Regular Tea Drinking on Iron Accumulation in Genetic Haemochromatosis." *Gut*, 1998; 43: 699–704.

INFLAMMATORY DISEASES

Devaraj, S., and I. Jialal. "Alpha Tocopherol Supplementation Decreases Serum C-Reactive Protein and Monocyte Interleukin-6 Levels in Normal Volunteers and Type 2 Diabetic Patients." *Free Radical Biology and Medicine*, 2000; 29:790–92.

Edmonds, S. E., P. G. Yinyard, R. Guo, et al. "Putative Analgesic Activity of Repeated Oral Doses of Vitamin E in the Treatment of Rheumatoid Arthritis. Results of a Prospective Placebo Controlled Double Blind Trial." *Annals of the Rheumatic Diseases*, 1997; 56:649–55.

Curtis, C. L., C. E. Hughes, C. R. Flannery, et al. "N-3 Fatty Acids Specifically Modulate Catabolic Factors Involved in Articular Cartilage Degradation." *Journal of Biological Chemistry*, 2000; 275:721–24.

Helmy, M., M. Shohayeb, M. H. Helmy, et al. "Antioxidants as Adjuvant Therapy in Rheumatoid Disease—a Preliminary Study." *Arzneimittel-Forschung/Drug Research*, 2001; 51:293–98.

Jenkinson, A. M., A. R. Collins, S. J. Duthie, et al. "The Effect of Increased Intakes of Polyunsaturated Fatty Acids and Vitamin E on DNA Damage in Human Lymphocytes." *FASEB Journal*, 1999; 13:2138–42.

Kornman, K. S., P. M. Martha, and G. W. Duff. "Genetic Variations and Inflammation: A Practical Nutrigenomics Opportunity." *Nutrition*, 2004; 20:44–49.

Lau, C. S., K. D. Morley, and J. J. F. Belch. "Effects of Fish Oil Supplementation on Non-Steroidal Anti-Inflammatory Drug Requirement in Patients with Mild Rheumatoid Arthritis—A Double-Blind Placebo Controlled Study." *British Journal of Rheumatology*, 1993; 32:982–89.

Linos, A., V. G. Kaklamani, E. Kaklamani, et al. "Dietary Factors in Relation to Rheumatoid Arthritis: A Role for Olive Oil and Cooked Vegetables." *American Journal of Clinical Nutrition*, 1999; 70:1077–82.

Liu, S., J. E. Manson, J. Buring, et al. "A High-Glycemic Diet in Relation to Plasma Levels of High-Sensitivity C-Reactive Protein in Middle-Aged Women." *American Journal of Epidemiology*, 2001; 153 (Suppl 11):S97.

Upritchard, J. E., W. H. F. Sutherland, and J. I. Mann. "Effect of Supplementation with Tomato Juice, Vitamin E, and Vitamin C on LDL Oxidation and Products of Inflammatory Activity in Type 2 Diabetes." *Diabetes Care*, 2000; 23:733–38.

Zurier, R. B., R. G. Rossetti, E. W. Jacobson, et al. "Gamma-Linolenic Acid Treatment of Rheumatoid Arthritis. A Randomized, Placebo-Controlled Study." *Arthritis and Rheumatism*, 1996; 11:1808–17.

OSTEOPOROSIS

Dimai, H. P., S. Porta, G. Wirmsberger, et al. "Daily Oral Magnesium Supplementation Suppresses Bone Turnover in Young Adult Males." *Journal of Clinical Endocrinol-*

ogy and Metabolism, 1998; 83:2742–48.

Guillemant, J., H.-T. Le, C. Accarie, et al. "Mineral Water as a Source of Dietary Calcium: Acute Effects on Parathyroid Function and Bone Resorption in Young Men." *American Journal of Clinical Nutrition*, 2000; 71:999–1002.

Hegarty, V. M., H. M. May, and K.-T. Khaw. "Tea Drinking and Bone Mineral Density in Older Women." *American Journal of Clinical Nutrition*, 2000; 71:1003–7.

Kim, G. S., C. H. Kim, J. Y. Park, et al. "Effects of Vitamin B$_{12}$ on Cell Proliferation and Cellular Alkaline Phosphatase Activity in Human Bone Marrow Stromal Osteoprogenitor Cells and UMR106 Osteoblastic Cells." *Metabolism*, 1996; 45:1443–46.

Mühlbauer, R. C., and F. Li. "Effect of Vegetables on Bone Metabolism." *Nature*, 1999; 401:343–44.

New, S. A., S. P. Robins, M. K. Campbell, et al. "Dietary Influences on Bone Mass and Bone Metabolism: Further Evidence of a Positive Link between Fruit and Vegetable Consumption and Bone Health. *American Journal of Clinical Nutrition*, 2000; 71:142–51.

Sokoll, L. J., S. L. Booth, M. E. O'Brien, et al. "Changes in Serum Osteocalcin, Plasma Phylloquinone, and Urinary Gamma-Carboxyglutamic Acid in Response to Altered Intakes of Dietary Phylloquinone in Human Subjects." *American Journal of Clinical Nutrition*, 1997; 65:779–84.

THE VITAMIN D QUANDARY

Bretherton-Watt, D., R. Given-Wilson, J. L. Mansi, et al. "Vitamin D Receptor Gene Polymorphisms Are Associated with Breast Cancer Risk in a UK Caucasian Population." *British Journal of Cancer*, 2001; 85:171–75.

Hayes, C. E. "Vitamn D: National Inhibitor of Multiple Sclerosis." *Proceedings of the Nutrition Society*, 2000; 59:531–35.

Hou, M. F., Y. C. Tien, G. T. Lin, et al. "Association of Vitamin D Receptor Gene Polymorphism with Sporadic Breast Cancer in Taiwanese Patients." *Breast Cancer Research and Treatment*, 2002; 74:1–7.

Ogata, E. "The Potential Use of Vitamin D Analogs in the Treatment of Cancer." *Calicified Tissue International*, 1997; 60:130–33.

Ortlepp, J. R., J. Lauscher, R. Hoffman, et al. "The Vitamin D Receptor Gene Variant Is Associated with the Prevalence of Type 2 Diabetes Mellitus and Coronary Artery Disease." *Diabetic Medicine*, 2001; 18:842–45.

Sheehan, D., T. Bennett, and K. D. Cashman. "An Assessment of Genetic Markers as Predictors of Bone Turnover in Healthy Adults." *Journal of Endocrinological Investigation*, 2001; 24:236–45.

———. "The Genetics of Osteoporosis: Vitamin D Receptor Gene Polymorphisms and Circulating Osteocalcin in Healthy Irish Adults." *Irish Journal of Medical Science*, 2001; 170:54–57.

Xu, Y., A. Shbiata, J. E. McNeal, et al. "Vitamin D Receptor Start Codon Polymorphisms (Fokl) and Prostate Cancer Progression." *Cancer Epidemiology Biomarkers and Prevention*, 2003; 12:23–27.

Zitterman, A., S. S. Schleithoff, G. Tenderich, et al. "Low Vitamin D Status: A Contributing Factor in the Pathogenesis of Congestive Heart Failure?" *Journal of the American College of Cardiology*, 2003; 41:105–12.

OBESITY AND TYPE 2 DIABETES

Anderson, R. A., N. Chen, N. A. Bryden, et al. "Elevated Intakes of Supplemental Chromium Improve Glucose and Insulin Variables in Individuals with Type 2 Diabetes." *Diabetes*, 1997; 46:1786–91.

de Vegt, F., J. M. Dekker, A. Jager, et al. "Relation of Impaired Fasting and Postload Glucose with Incident Type 2 Diabetes in a Dutch Population. The Hoorn Study." *Journal of the American Medical Association*, 2001; 285:2109–13.

Diamond, J. "The Double Puzzle of Diabetes." *Nature*, 2003; 423:599–602.

Khan, A., M. Safdar, M. M. A. Khan, et al. "Cinnamon Improves Glucose and Lipids of People with Type 2 Diabetes." *Diabetes Care*, 2003; 26:3215–18.

Khaw, K. T., N. Wareham, R. Luben, et al. "Glycated Hemoglobin, Diabetes, and Mortality in Men in Norfolk Cohort of European Prospective Investigations of Cancer and Nutrition (EPIC-Norfolk)." *British Medical Journal*, 2001; 322;1–6.

Johnston, C. S., C. M. Kim, and A. J. Buller. "Vinegar Improves Insulin Sensitivity to a High-Carbohydrate Meal in Subjects with Insulin Resistance or Type 2 Diabetes." *Diabetes Care*, 2004; 27:281–82.

Ludwig, D. S. "The Glycemic Index. Physiological Mechanisms Relating to Obesity, Diabetes, and Cardiovascular Disease." *Journal of the American Medical Association*, 2002; 287:2414–23.

McLeod, M. N., B. N. Gaynes, and R. N. Golden. "Chromium Potentiation of Antidepressant Pharmacology for Dysthymic Disorder in 5 Patients." *Journal of Clinical Psychiatry*, 1999; 60:237–40.

———, and R. N. Golden. "Chromium Treatment of Depression." *International Journal of Neuropsychopharmacology*; 2000; 3:311–14.

Velussi, M., A. M. Cernigoi, A. D. De Monte, et al. "Long-Term (12 Months) Treatment with an Antioxidant Drug (Silymarin) Is Effective on Hyperinsulinemia, Exogenous Insulin Need and Malondialdehyde Levels in Cirrhotic Diabetic Patients." *Journal of Hepatology*, 1997; 26:871–79.

Parkinson's Disease

Chen, H., S. M. Zhang, M. A. Hernan, et al. "Diet and Parkinson's disease: A Potential Role of Dairy Products in Men." *Annals of Neurology*, 2002; 52:793–801.

Ciccone, C. D. "Free-Radical Toxicity and Antioxidant Medications in Parkinson's Disease." *Physical Therapy*, 1998; 78:313–19.

Duan, W., B. Ladenheim, R. G. Cutler, et al. "Dietary Folate Deficiency and Elevated Homocysteine Levels Endanger Dopaminergic Neurons in Models of Parkinson's Disease." *Journal of Neurochemistry*, 2002; 80:101–10.

Shults, C. W., D. Oakes, K. Kieburtz, et al. "Effects of Coenzyme Q10 in Early Parkinson Disease. Evidence of Slowing of the Functional Decline." *Archives of Neurology*, 2002; 59:1541–50.

Zhang, S. M., M. A. Hernan, H. Chen, et al. "Intakes of Vitamins E and C, Carotenoids, Vitamin Supplements, and PD Risk." *Neurology*, 2002; 59:1161–69.

Pyroluria

Jackson, J. A., H. D. Riordan, S. Neathery, et al. "Urinary Pyrroles in Health and Disease." *Journal of Orthomolecular Medicine*, 1997; 12:96–98.

———. "Urinary Pyrroles Revisited." *Journal of Orthomolecular Medicine*, 2001; 16:47–48.

Sickle-Cell Anemia

Kennedy, T. S., E. B. Fung, D. A. Kawchak, et al. "Red Blood Cell Folate and Serum Vitamin B_{12} Status in Children with Sickle Cell Disease." *Journal of Pediatric Hematology/Oncology*, 2001; 23:165–69.

Marwah, S. S., D. Wheelwright, A. Blann, et al. "Vitamin E Correlates Inversely with

Non-Transferrin-Bound Iron in Sickle Cell Disease." *British Journal of Haematology*, 2001; 114:917–19.

Ohnishi, S. T., T. Ohnishi, G. B. Ogunmola. "Green Tea Extract and Aged Garlic Extract Inhibit Anion Transport and Sickle Cell Dehydration In Vitro." *Blood Cells, Molecules, and Diseases*, 2001; 27:148–57.

———. "Sickle Cell Anemia: A Potential Nutritional Approach for a Molecular Disease." *Nutrition*, 2000; 16:330–38.

Shukla. P., S. M. Graham, A. Borgstein, et al. "Sickle Cell Disease and Vitamin E Deficiency in Children in Developing Countries." *Transactions of the Royal Society of Tropical Medicine*, 2000; 94:109.

SKIN AGING AND WRINKLES

Fisher, G. J., S. Kang, J. Varani, et al. "Mechanisms of Photoaging and Chronological Skin Aging." *Archives of Dermatology*, 2002; 138:1462–70.

Eberlein-König, B., M. Placzek, and B. Pryzybilla. "Protective Effect against Sunburn of Combined Systemic Ascorbic Acid (Vitamin C) and D-A-Tocopherol (Vitamin E)." *Journal of the American Academy of Dermatology*, 1998; 38:45–48.

Heinrich, U., C. Gartner, M. Wiebusch, et al. "Supplementation with Beta-Carotene or a Similar Amount of Mixed Carotenoids Protects Humans from UV-Induced Erythema." *Journal of Nutrition*, 2003; 133:98–101.

Lee, J., S. Jiang, N. Levine, et al. "Carotenoid Supplementation Reduces Erythema in Human Skin after Simulated Solar Radiation Exposure." *Proceedings of the Society for Experimental Biology and Medicine*, 2000; 223:170–74.

Purba, M., A. Kouris-Blazos, N. Wattanapenpaiboon, et al. "Skin Wrinkling: Can Food Make a Difference?" *Journal of the American College of Nutrition*, 2001; 20:71–80.

Saliou, C., G. Rimbach, H. Moini, et al. "Solar Ultraviolet-Induced Erythema in Human Skin and Nuclear Factor-Kappa-B-Dependent Gene Expression in Keratinocytes Are Modulated by a French Maritime Pine Bark Extract." *Free Radical Biology and Medicine*, 2001; 30;154–60.

Thiele, J., and P. Elsner. *Oxidants and Antioxidants in Cutaneous Biology*. Basel: Karger, 2001.

Trekli, M. C., G. Riss, R. Goralczyk, et al. "Beta-Carotene Suppresses UVA-Induced HO-1 Gene Expression in Cultured FEK4." *Free Radical Biology and Medicine*, 2003; 34:456–64.

INDEX

antioxidants (*continued*)
  functions of, 6, 68–72
  inflammatory diseases and, 69, 74, 191
  Parkinson's disease and, 201
  skin care and, 206–208
  synergy, 72
  UV-ray exposure, wrinkles, and, 206–208
anxiety, 141, 147, 152
APOE E4 gene, cardiovascular disease and, 154, 174, 176
apoptosis, 70–71, 167
appetite, 145
apple cider vinegar, 199
arachidonic acid, 175
arginine, 66–67
arrowroot as sauce thickener, 124
arthritis, 147
Artichoke Hearts and Dijon Sauce, Shrimp with, 125
asparagine, 113
Asparagus, Simple Baked, 129
asthma, 10, 189
Atkins diet, 97–98
Avocado and Chicken Omelette, 133

bananas, 103
  and Nut Butter, Fresh, 135
Barrett's esophagus, 79–80
B-complex vitamins, 22, 37, 150, 160, 167–168, 174, 184, 186. See also *specific vitamins*
  DNA methylation and, 61–65
  DNA repair and, 6, 57–65
  supplement guidelines, 56, 67
Beal, Dr. M. Flint, 55
Beck, Melinda, 79, 178
Bellanti, Dr. Joseph, 55–56, 186
Benjamin, Dr. Jonathan, 151
beta-amyloid protein, 74, 159, 160
beta-carotene, 68, 71, 81–82, 173, 201, 207, 208
beverages, 107–108, 120, 150, 207
bioenergetics, 41–43
bioflavonoids. See flavonoids
birth defects, 14–15, 60–61, 142, 162–166. See also *specific birth defects*

the gene connection, 163–164
what happens, 162–163
what you can do, 164–166
Bjelland, Dr. Ingvar, 142
blindness, 195
bloodletting, 188
blood pressure, 45, 77
bone density, 36, 156, 191–194. See also osteoporosis
brain, the
  antidepressants and, 146
  antioxidants and, 69
  stress and, 147, 148–149
  structure, behaviors that modify genes and, 144–146
brain cancer, childhood, 163, 166
BRCA1 and BRCA2 genes, breast cancer and, 154, 169, 170
breads, whole-wheat, 112
breakfast recipes, 132–134
breast cancer, 71, 82, 85, 169–170, 172, 194, 197
  BRCA1 and BRCA2 genes, 154, 169, 170
  CHEK2 gene, 169
Brody, Dr. Stuart, 151
brown rice, 106–107, 120
  Seafood and, 124–125
burgers
  Chicken, with Romano Cheese and Olives/or Shiitake Mushrooms, 130
  Turkey, Simple, 130–131
butter, 105

caffeine, 150
calcium, 192–193, 194
calorie restriction, 32–33
cancer, 32, 48, 114, 167–173, 189, 196, 204. See also *specific types of cancer*
  antioxidants and, 69–70, 84, 85, 86, 173
  coenzyme Q10 and, 46, 172
  damaged DNA and, 12, 16
  DNA methylation and, 61–62
  DNA-repair efficiency and, 26
  folic acid and, 167, 171–172
  the gene connection, 168–170

ABOUT THE AUTHOR

Jack Challem, known as The Nutrition Reporter, is a leading health and medical writer and a regular contributor to *GreatLife, Let's Live, Alternative Medicine, Body & Soul, Natural Health, Modern Maturity,* and many other consumer and health magazines. His scientific articles have been published in *Free Radical Biology and Medicine,* the *Journal of Orthomolecular Medicine, Medical Hypotheses,* and other journals. Challem is also the author of John Wiley & Sons' *The Inflammation Syndrome* and the lead author of *Syndrome X.*

Printed in the USA
CPSIA information can be obtained
at www.ICGtesting.com
JSHW012014140824
68134JS00025B/2415